ESSENTIALS OF HEALTH PROMOTION

Brent Alexander

ALLIED HEALTH PRESS

Essentials of Health Promotion

Author: **Brent Alexander**

Allied Health Press
4164 Lakeshore Road
Burlington ON L7L 1A4
Canada
www.alliedhealthpress.com
Email: orders@arclereducation.com

ISBN: 978-1-77956-765-9

ABOUT THE AUTHOR

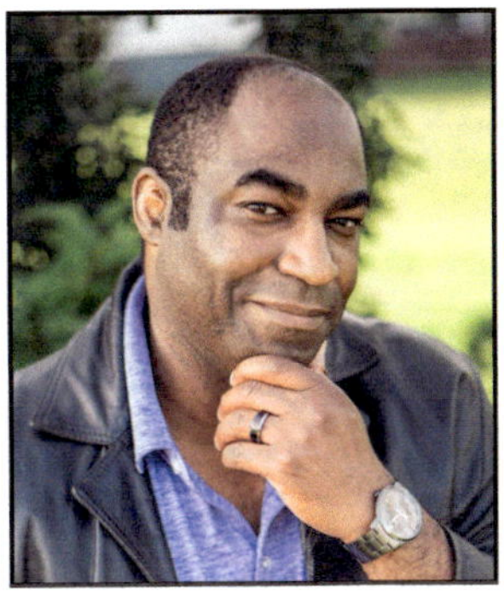

Brent Alexander is a dedicated, senior level, healthcare and life science advisor with over 14 years of medical research and healthcare consulting experience. He is skilled in strategic thinking, data analysis & interpretation, project management, and building relationships. Brent has effectively planned, executed, and evaluated several major medical research projects for organizations such as Suncor Energy Inc., Calgary Flames Hockey Organization, and Own the Podium. Brent has an intrinsic love for science and has expanded on this through gaining academic accolades in maternal/child health and perinatal physiology, as well as in the chronobiological and physiological principles of sleep medicine. Since completing a Masters degree in Medical Science, Brent has previously managed a role as the Clinical Research Coordinator at the Centre for Sleep and Human Performance, a College of Physicians and Surgeons of Alberta, and American Academy of Sleep Medicine accredited sleep centre in Calgary, Alberta. Currently, he holds two positions within Alberta Health Services – _Brent is the Senior Advisor for Public Health, Calgary Zone, providing integration of technology and quality improvement alignment with the clinical operations of immunization and public health programs. He is also a Tissue Specialist with the Southern Alberta Tissue Program where he uses his laboratory experience to expertly assist in the surgical recovery, processing, preservation and distribution of donor tissues that are used for banking, transplantation, and research procedures help improve the quality of life for Albertans. Brent is also an accomplished writer and editor. He has authored and co-authored several abstracts and peer reviewed articles on fever & pregnancy, jet lag & travel fatigue management in elite athletes, and sleep & long-term athletic development (LTAD). In his down time, Brent enjoys staying active through sports and enjoying the outdoors with his wife and son.

Brief Table of Contents

Detailed Table of Contents

LIST OF FIGURES

PREFACE

Health promotion is an essential component of public health that seeks to enhance the overall welfare of individuals and communities. It includes a broad array of tactics and measures aimed at averting illness, encouraging beneficial habits, and improving overall well-being. The field of health promotion is in a perpetual state of evolution as new research and evidence-based practices continue to emerge on a regular basis.

The significance of this book lies in its capacity to address the increasing demand for efficient health promotion initiatives in contemporary society. Given the rising prevalence of chronic diseases and health problems associated with lifestyle choices, there is a pressing need for easily accessible and scientifically supported information to assist individuals and organizations in promoting health and preventing diseases. This book tackles the lack of information by providing a comprehensive analysis of important ideas, theories, and practical applications in the field of health promotion.

The motivation for this book stems from a desire to equip individuals with the knowledge and expertise needed to make well-informed decisions about their health. The book aims to inspire readers to improve their health and well-being by offering a variety of strategies and interventions.

This book will appeal to a diverse audience including students, healthcare professionals, public health practitioners, and policymakers. It will be a valuable resource for students studying health promotion, public health, nursing, or related fields. The book offers practical insights that will benefit healthcare professionals seeking to enhance their knowledge and skills in health promotion; additionally, it will be a valuable resource for public health practitioners and policymakers seeking evidence-based approaches to improve population-level health.

Readers will benefit from this book by gaining a deeper understanding of the principles and methodologies of health promotion. By exploring key concepts such as health behavior modification, social factors influencing health, and health communication, individuals will acquire the necessary expertise to develop and implement successful health promotion initiatives.

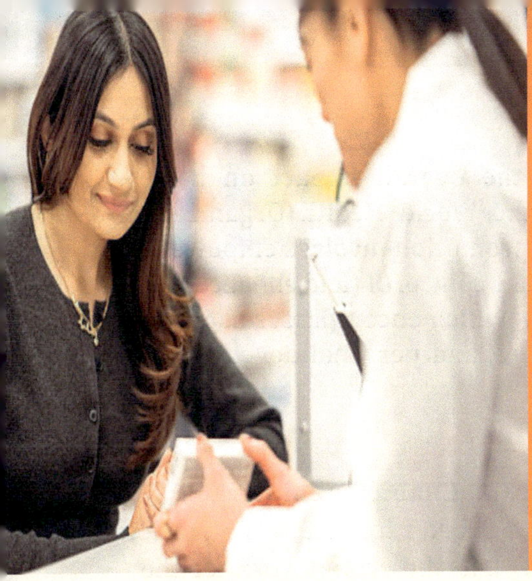

Chapter 1

INTRODUCTION TO HEALTH PROMOTION

Contents

1.1. A Brief Overview on Health Promotion

According to the World Health Organization, health encompasses more than just the absence of disease. It is a comprehensive state of physical, mental, and emotional well-being. Promotion is an activity that provides support or encouragement for a cause or aim. Health Promotion involves empowering individuals to take control of their health and make improvements. This perspective expands beyond an emphasis on individual actions to encompass a broad array of social and environmental interventions (Figure 1.1).

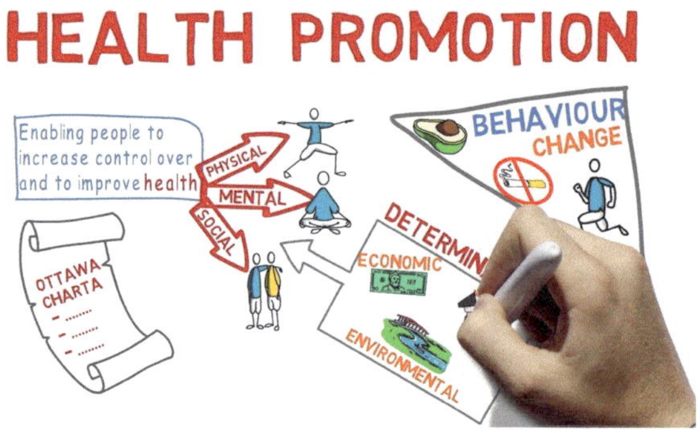

Figure 1.1. *An illustration of health promotion.*

Source: Global Health with Greg Martin (2022).

Health promotion is an essential component of public health as it enables governments, communities, and individuals to effectively address and resolve significant health concerns (Haugan & Eriksson, 2021). Various measures are implemented to establish policies, create conducive environments, and motivate communities to take action, and strategic efforts are made to improve these three stakeholder's ability to communicate and cooperate together.

Health promotion is a dynamic process that extends beyond the individual to encompass the people and environment around them...as well as the larger system. At the heart of this endeavor lies a profound sense of purpose – to empower individuals to reclaim their health and achieve wellness. According to Haugan and Eriksson (2021), health promotion encompasses a wide range of dimensions. The fundamental goal of health promotion is to mitigate risks and foster positive health behaviors.

1.1.1. The Essence of Health Promotion

Health promotion has evolved beyond education alone and now encompasses a wide range of changes that span from health education to health behavior. The approach here is to consider the broader perspective, recognizing how various factors are interconnected and contribute to the overall impact on health. According to the World Health Organization (WHO), health promotion involves empowering individuals to take control of (and enhance) their own well-being, which encompasses aspects of safety, healthcare, and personal development.

1.1.2. Key Strategies

- **Advocate, Enable, Mediate:** The Ottawa Charter for Health Promotion (1986) laid the groundwork for the global health promotion initiatives that exist today. Three fundamental strategies were identified:
    - **Advocate:** The importance of emphasizing and encouraging elements of wellness. It is important to promote policies that create a positive environment for well-being. This involves advocating for the necessary environments and practices to support well-being. Consider the instances when campaigns establish smoke-free zones, promote physical activity, and encourage healthy diets.
    - **Enable:** Promote equal access to healthcare for all. It is essential that every individual is afforded equal opportunities to experience optimal health. Promote and strengthen individual, societal, and governmental accomplishments in addressing issues and surmounting obstacles.
- **Mediate:** Collaboration across sectors is crucial for effective mediation. A successful public health initiative requires the collaboration of various stakeholders, including

government, civil society, academia, and businesses. Mediation fosters a sense of calm, encourages a cooperative mindset, and ultimately leads to resolution.

1.1.3. Beyond Individual Behavior

Health promotion extends beyond individual decisions and encompasses a broader scope. It acknowledges the influence of various factors on one's health:

- **Social Determinants:** Income, level of education, place of living, and social support all play significant roles in determining one's overall health. It is crucial to consider how to effectively tackle these issues within the realm of health promotion.
- **Environmental Interventions:** Consider the concept of constructing in pedestrian areas, allocating spaces for greenspaces, and ensuring the preservation of clean water. These environmental changes play a vital role in sustaining our bodies.

1.1.4. Understanding Health

An essential aspect of fostering empowerment involves educating individuals on health literacy. Understanding health goes beyond just reading leaflets. It involves analyzing data, collaborating with healthcare institutions, and making informed decisions. Individuals who possess a comprehensive understanding of health matters are inclined to proactively implement measures to protect and enhance their overall quality of life.

1.1.5. Creating Healthy Settings

When considering environmental interventions, it is important to acknowledge that the places where individuals reside, work, and engage in recreational activities have a profound impact on their overall well-being. Let's take into consideration:

- **Schools:** Within schools, it is important to emphasize the significance of daily exercise along with being mindful of a student's mental well-being and maintenance of a nutritious diet.
- **Workplaces:** All workplaces should consider implementing exercise and restoration classes, incorporating ergonomic design, and providing stress management resources.
- **Communities:** Communities play a crucial role in ensuring the provision of safe drinking water, maintaining open health facilities, and fostering positive relationships among individuals. These factors are essential for the well-being and harmony of society.

Health promotion is not dependent on any one individual for its implementation; rather, it is a collective responsibility that is shared among many. When considering discussions on health, one cannot help but envision a future of abundance, where individuals possess the tools to shape their own futures. By actively engaging in health promotion, individuals can make significant strides towards achieving universal healthcare for all.

1.2. Historical Overview of Health Promotion

Health promotion has a rich history that can be traced back to various ancient civilizations. Among these, the Greeks stand out as having a particularly noteworthy influence. Their innovative approach to health established the basis for modern health promotion. Here is a historical tour that explores the impact of their wisdom on the development of wellbeing, as discussed by Raphael (2008).

- **Eliminating the Paranormal Phenomena:** In the sixth and fourth century B.C., the Greeks were able to liberate health and illness from the metaphysical constraints that had previously confined them. Illnesses were no longer attributed solely to supernatural forces or divine wrath. Instead, they embraced a physiocratic philosophy that is rooted in the study of human behavior and natural phenomena.
- **Key Concepts from Classical Greece:** The Greeks introduced significant concepts that continue to hold relevance in modern times:
    - **Comprehensive Perspective:** The connection between wellbeing and the climate was not always separate. The balance between internal and external factors was truly exceptional. It was evident to the Greeks that the state of wellbeing was intricately linked to both the physical environment and social contexts.
    - **Determinants of Wellbeing:** When considering the factors that contribute to overall wellbeing, both physical and social determinants were taken into account. Various factors, such as sustenance, cleanliness, and the local community, have a significant impact on overall well-being.
    - **Strengthening:** The Greeks had a strong belief in actively involving individuals and communities. They established a framework that emphasized fairness and inclusivity, with a strong focus on promoting well-being and professional growth.
    - **Steady Conditions:** Recognizing the importance of environmental factors, they advocated for favorable conditions that promote well-being.
    - **Naturalistic Medication:** Their clinical perspective shifted towards a more naturalistic and humanistic approach. They valued harmony, balance, and self-control.
- **Pythagoreans and the Pursuit of Harmony:** The Pythagoreans emphasized the importance of friendship, balance, and unity. It was believed that by controlling irritation (whether through diet, behavior, or emotions) one could improve their overall health. Their core values revolved around cleanliness, balance, and tranquility.
- **Plato's Perspective on Wellbeing:** Plato, the logician, envisioned wellbeing as a state of harmony with the universe. In Plato's belief, it is crucial to prioritize fulfillment and happiness. He had a broad perspective that extended beyond the physical realm, encompassing mental and profound well-being.
- **Inheritance and Current Pertinence:** The ancient Greeks laid

the foundations for the advancement of well-being. Their expertise lies in the Ottawa Sanction for Wellbeing Advancement. They understood that well-being is interconnected with social, environmental, and personal factors. Our heritage continues to shape our pursuit of prosperity in the 21st century.

1.3. Influence Beyond the Greeks

Aside from Greek influence, several examples of health promotion approaches have emerged from the rich traditions of other cultures around the world including India, China, Egypt, and the Hebrews.

- **Indian Systems of Medicine:** Ancient Indian culture encompasses a wide range of traditional healing practices that have been passed down through generations. These systems, such as Ayurveda and Siddha, are deeply rooted in holistic approaches to health and well-being. They emphasize the balance of mind, body, and spirit, and believe in the power of natural remedies and therapies.
- **Traditional Chinese Medicine (2700 BC):** Emphasizes the importance of cleanliness, diet, hydrotherapy, and vaccination.
- **Traditional Egyptian Medicine:** In 200 BC, the Egyptians made significant advancements in their society. They implemented efficient water collection systems, improved garbage disposal methods, and implemented practices to prevent the spread of diseases. They emphasized the importance of using mosquito nets, maintaining good hygiene through frequent bathing, and practicing moderation when it comes to alcohol consumption.
- **Hebrew Insight:** The Mosaic Regulation emphasized the importance of rest, cleanliness, and avoiding destructive practices. The Code of Hammurabi and the Mosaic Regulation are two ancient legal systems that have had a significant impact on the development of law.
- **Code of Hammurabi:** The Code of Hammurabi covers various aspects such as preventing sickness, managing waste disposal, and isolating individuals with contagious diseases.
- **Mosaic Regulation:** Emphasized the importance of taking regular rest days for overall well-being, following dietary guidelines, and being aware of the risks associated with consuming pork.

The ancient Greeks ignited a spark that continues to illuminate the path of health promotion. Promoting wellbeing goes beyond individual choices, it involves creating prosperous societies. By intertwining ancient wisdom with modern scientific knowledge, one can construct a reality in which prosperity thrives – a world that echoes the harmonious ideals of Pythagoras and Plato.

1.4. Theoretical Frameworks of Health Promotion

Theory can be described as a collection of concepts, definitions, and propositions that aim to provide explanations or predictions for events or situations by illustrating the relationships between variables. Theoretical approaches are employed to analyze solutions for the questions of "why", "what", and "how" medical issues should be addressed. They analyze the concept of designated health behaviors by seeking answers to these questions. The role of theory in public health is crucial. It provides justifications for individuals' choices regarding their health behaviors, guides planners in determining their objectives before developing public health programs, and offers strategies for reaching target audiences and making a meaningful impact.

Winett, R. A. (1995) categorizes the theories and models used for health promotion into the following:

- **Health Belief Model:** The health belief model serves as a theoretical framework for guiding health promotion programs. This concept is utilized to provide explanations and forecasts for individual shifts in health behaviors. This model is widely utilized in the field of health behavior research and analysis. The Health Belief Model (HBM) explores how individuals perceive the potential threat of a health problem, including their susceptibility to it and the severity of the problem. It also considers the benefits of taking action to avoid the threat, as well as the factors that influence their decision to act. These factors include barriers that may hinder their actions, cues that may prompt them to take action, and their own self-efficacy in carrying out the necessary steps. The model emphasizes the importance of individual beliefs about health conditions in predicting individual health-related behaviors. There are several factors that have an impact on health behaviors.
    - **Perceived Susceptibility:** This refers to an individual's perception of the threat of sickness or disease.
    - **Perceived Severity:** This refers to an individual's belief regarding the potential consequences of a particular situation or event.
    - **Potential Positive Benefits of Action:** These are often considered when evaluating the perceived advantages.
    - **Cues to Action:** One important aspect to consider when it comes to taking action is the cues that prompt us to do so. These cues can come in the form of perceived barriers that may hinder our progress, or exposure to factors that motivate us to take action. Both of these elements play a crucial role in determining whether or not we will actually take the necessary steps towards our goals.
    - **Self-Efficacy:** This refers to an individual's confidence in their ability to succeed.
- **Transtheoretical Model:** The transtheoretical model (TTM) is a widely recognized framework that helps individuals understand and navigate the process of behavior change. It is an advanced conceptual framework used to understand the adoption and maintenance of intentional health behaviors.

TTM identifies five key phases of progress: precontemplation, contemplation, readiness, action, and maintenance. These phases represent the transient and influential aspects of change.

TTM and its impact on physical activity is a process that occurs in stages over time, with individuals engaging in different mental and social cycles at various points of progress. These cycles serve as the building blocks of change. Individuals will also consider the pros and cons of engaging in physical activity. As individuals move through the stages of adjusting their work propensity, they will experience an increase in self-reliance. TTM has been widely utilized to determine active work correlations such as instances when individuals begin to consider the benefits and drawbacks of real-world employment. It has been shown that as individuals navigate the various stages of adjusting their work propensity, they typically experience an enhanced sense of self-efficacy.

- **The Theory of Reasoned Action/ Planned Behavior:** The focus of this theory is the development of a framework for understanding two sets of factors: perspectives – which refer to positive or negative feelings related to achieving a goal; and emotional standards – which are specific descriptions of an individual's perception of an object's ability to achieve those goals.

For instance, when it comes to tobacco use, planned behavior theory suggests that an individual's intentions to engage in a certain behavior are not fixed and can be influenced by various factors, including:

  - **Perspectives:** An individual's beliefs regarding the qualities and outcomes of using tobacco (or quitting), as assessed by their evaluations of these qualities and outcomes.
  - **Emotional Standards:** An individual's beliefs about the approval or disapproval of tobacco use by significant others, influenced by their motivation to conform to these desires.
  - **Social Control:** This refers to an individual's perception of their ability to regulate their tobacco use, taking into account the presence or absence of factors that may hinder or support their efforts to quit.

- **Social Cognitive Theory:** This is one of the most comprehensive models in health promotion that addresses both the underlying factors of health behavior and the strategies for promoting change, focusing on the interplay between individuals and their environment. The fundamental components of social cognitive theory include reciprocal determinism, environmental influences, personal factors, and behavioral outcomes.
- **Ecological Models:** This model explores the intricate relationships and interconnections among various factors at different levels of a health problem. This concept focuses on how individuals engage with their surroundings, both in terms of the physical world and the social and cultural aspects (Figure 1.2).

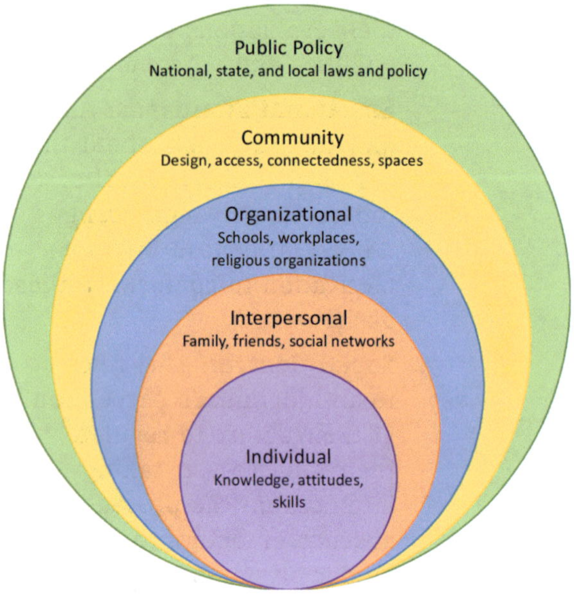

Figure 1.2. *Ecological models of health promotion.*

Source: Fry et al. (2022).

Ecological models acknowledge the various factors that can impact health behaviors. These include:

- The influence of intrapersonal or individual factors: These factors encompass a range of elements, including knowledge, attitudes, beliefs, and personality traits. Understanding how these factors shape behavior is crucial in gaining a comprehensive understanding of human actions.
- Institutional and organizational factors: These play a crucial role in shaping healthy behaviors. These factors encompass a wide range of elements, such as rules, regulations, policies, and informal structures. Understanding how these factors influence behavior is essential for promoting a healthy environment.
- Community factors: They play a significant role in shaping healthy behaviors. These factors include the formal and informal social norms that exist among individuals, groups, or organizations. They have the power to either limit or enhance the adoption of healthy behaviors.
- Public policy factors: They encompass a wide range of regulations and laws at the local, state, and federal levels. These policies play a crucial role in governing and supporting various health actions, such as early detection, control, and management.

1.5. Principles of Health Promotion

As Rootman, (2001) explains, there are several principles that serve as a framework for developing strategies, policies, and actions aimed at enhancing health on individual, community, and global scales.

- **Strengthening**: This is an approach that aims to empower individuals to manage decisions and actions that affect their well-being.
- **Participative**: This refers to a situation where individuals actively engage in the process of navigation. Examining the various effects on overall well-being and the correlation between these factors.
- **Impartial**: Ensuring fairness and impartiality in delivering quality results for valued clients.
- **Intersectoral:** This refers to the collaboration and coordination between different offices and associations that are relevant to a particular field or issue.

- **Feasible**: Ensuring that the results of health promotion activities are sustainable in the long term is crucial.
- **Multi System**: addressing different technique regions such as projects and strategy.

The World Wellbeing Association played a significant role in driving the efforts for health promotion in the 1980s, with the publication of the Ottawa Charter in 1986. Wellbeing promotion occurs at five key levels, according to the proposal.

1. Creating individual abilities
2. Establishing steady conditions
3. Fortifying people group activity
4. Creating public approach
5. Re-arranging the wellbeing adm inistrations

1.6. The Importance of Health Promotion Among Young People

1.6.1. Developing Personal Skills

Through a wide range of programs and activities, youth organizations have a positive impact on the personal development of young people. These include health education, providing information, and fostering the growth of important skills such as self-esteem, self-efficacy, communication, negotiation, life skills, and motivation. Developing these skills has a significant impact on one's overall health.

1.6.2. Creating Supportive Environments

This is an essential aspect of fostering positive growth and development. It involves establishing a framework that encourages individuals to thrive and reach their full potential. By implementing strategies that promote inclusivity, empathy, and understanding, we can cultivate an atmosphere where everyone feels valued and supported. Youth organizations play a crucial role in fostering safe and supportive environments for young people and staff. These environments encourage open discussions about health issues and promote healthy behaviors. By offering healthy food options in cafeterias, providing nutritious snacks for after-school clubs, creating smoke-free spaces, implementing anti-bullying policies, and offering adolescent-friendly health services, these organizations make it easier for individuals to make healthier choices.

1.6.3. Strengthening Community Action

One way to enhance community action is by fostering a sense of unity and collaboration among its members. By encouraging individuals to come together and work towards a common goal, we can create a stronger and more resilient community. This can be achieved through various means such as organizing community events, promoting volunteerism, and supporting local initiatives. By strengthening community action

By fostering collaborations and forming alliances with various organizations and sectors in the community, youth organizations have the opportunity to enhance their capabilities and make a positive impact on the overall health of the community. This, in turn, enables them to better support the health needs of their target groups residing within the community. For instance, when community action is strengthened, youth organizations are well positioned to deliver high-impact parent programs and work in partnership with healthy towns initiatives that provide effective results.

1.6.4. Delivering Health Public Policy

By implementing health-related policies, youth organizations showcase their commitment to evidence-based practice. These policies (such as those addressing sexual health and substance use) play a crucial role in supporting their operational practices. In addition, youth organizations play a crucial role in raising awareness and advocating for public policy development and change to support their health-related initiatives and the well-being of their target groups. One example of this is a regional or national alcohol policy.

1.6.5. Reorienting Health Services

Youth organizations play a crucial role in promoting and advocating for the development and provision of health services that cater to the specific needs of young people. For instance, they are actively involved in raising awareness and advocating for the establishment of adolescent-friendly health services.

1.7. Levels of Prevention in Health Promotion

Prevention encompasses a diverse array of activities referred to as "interventions" that are designed to mitigate risks or hazards to health (Ureda & Yates, 2005). Researchers and health experts often discuss three categories of prevention: primary, secondary, and tertiary (Figure 1.3).

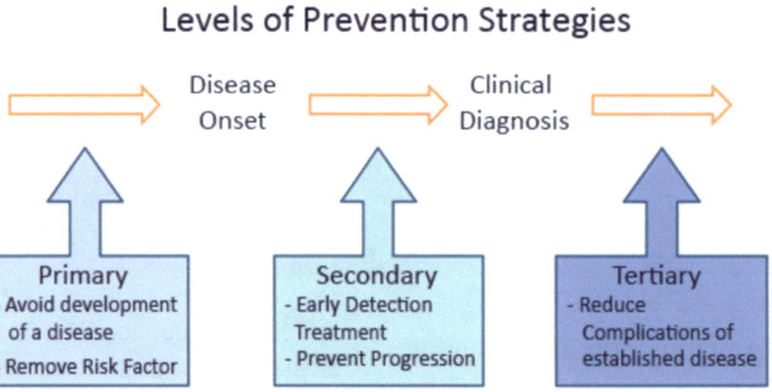

Figure 1.3. *Public health approach to promotion.*

Source: Preventive Services | PCORE (2020).

1.7.1. Primary Prevention

This refers to the proactive measures taken to prevent the occurrence of a particular disease or health condition. It involves implementing strategies and interventions that target the root causes and risk factors associated with the condition. By focusing on prevention rather than treatment, primary prevention aims to reduce the overall burden of disease and promote better health.

As Ureda and Yates (2005) explain, primary prevention is focused on preventing illness or injury before it occurs. This is achieved by proactively addressing potential sources of harm or danger that can lead to infection or injury, modifying unhealthy or risky behaviors that may contribute to illness or injury, and enhancing safeguards against illness or injury in the event of exposure. One approach to address safety concerns is through the implementation of regulations and authorizations. These measures can be used to boycott or control the use of hazardous products (e.g., asbestos), or to mandate the adoption of safe practices, like the use of seat belts and bicycle helmets. Learning about sound and safe habits, such as maintaining a healthy diet, exercising regularly, and avoiding smoking, as well as the importance of getting vaccinated against infectious diseases are key elements of primary prevention.

1.7.2. Secondary Prevention

This is an important aspect to consider in healthcare. Secondary prevention involves strategies to mitigate the impact of an infection or injury that has already occurred. This is accomplished by promptly recognizing and addressing infection or injury, in order to prevent further progression or slow its advancement. It also involves empowering individuals with strategies to prevent reinjury or recurrence, and implementing programs to restore individuals to their original health and functionality, with the aim of preventing long-term complications. There are different types of models that are used in secondary prevention.

- Ordinary tests, which are commonly used to detect various illnesses.
- Screening tests, which are specifically designed to identify diseases in their earliest stages. For instance, mammograms are a type of screening test that is used to detect breast cancer.
- Routine interventions, such as the daily use of low-dose ibuprofen and the implementation of diet and exercise programs can effectively prevent future respiratory failures or strokes. These measures also facilitate the safe return of injured or ill workers to their jobs.

1.7.3. Tertiary Prevention

This refers to the stage of intervention that focuses on minimizing the impact of a disease or condition that has already occurred. It involves strategies and treatments aimed at preventing further complications and improving the quality of life for individuals who are already affected. Tertiary prevention focuses on mitigating the long-term consequences of a persistent illness or injury. The goal is to assist individuals in managing long-term, and often complex medical conditions and injuries. Tertiary prevention also aims at improving people's ability to function, enhance their quality of life, and optimize their future. Some examples of tertiary preventions offered in most places include cardiovascular or stroke recovery programs, as well as ongoing infection management programs for conditions such as diabetes, arthritis, and depression. There are also support programs that encourage individuals to share strategies for successful professional rehabilitation initiatives aimed at retraining workers for new positions once they have recovered.

1.8. Role of Health Promotion in Public Health

Health promotion is an essential component of public health, as it plays a critical role in improving well-being, preventing diseases, and fostering healthier populations (Potvin & Jones, 2011). Health promotion plays a crucial role in enhancing the overall health of individuals, communities, and societies. It tackles various health concerns through a range of comprehensive strategies.

Health promotion takes into account a comprehensive perspective on health that goes beyond simply managing diseases. According to the World Health Organization (WHO), health promotion involves empowering individuals to take charge of their own health and improve it. According to Potvin and Jones (2011), the roles of health promotion in public health are as follows:

- **Implementing Comprehensive Public Policies:** Health promotion emphasizes the importance of implementing policies that create supportive environments. The impact of these policies extends beyond the health sector, affecting education, income, and living conditions. Health promotion plays a crucial role in ensuring that decisions made across different sectors have a positive impact on health outcomes. It achieves this by focusing on strengthening governance and making healthy choices more accessible and affordable for everyone.
- **Empowering Individuals and Communities:** Enhancing one's health literacy empowers individuals to actively engage in their own health journey. It is crucial for citizens to have a comprehensive understanding of health information in order to effectively advocate for their own well-being and ensure that governments are held responsible for public health.
- **Giving People and Communities More Power:** Community participation is crucial for health promotion to thrive. When communities actively engage and get involved, the impact of health promotion is greatly enhanced. Healthier populations are achieved through the combined efforts of communities, initiatives that are based on community involvement, and a sense of shared responsibility.
- **Creating Healthy Environments:** An important aspect of promoting health is the focus on creating healthy environments. These environments can include schools, workplaces, neighborhoods, and healthcare facilities. Through the promotion of healthy eating, raising awareness about mental health, and encouraging physical activity, these environments contribute to the overall well-being of individuals.
- **Health for All, a Global Commitment:** The World Health Organization (WHO) plays a crucial role in promoting health across all Sustainable Development Goals (SDGs). The main goal of SDGs is to guarantee the health and well-being of all individuals, without leaving anyone behind. According to the World Health Organization, the goal is to improve the health and well-being of an additional 1 billion people by 2023.
- **A Roadmap for Change: the Shanghai Declaration:** The 9th Global Conference on Health Promotion, which took place in Shanghai in 2016, highlighted the significant links between health promotion and the Sustainable Development Goals of the 2030

Agenda. To expedite country action on the SDGs, it emphasized the need for bold political interventions.

- **The Potential for Transformation:** This is a fascinating aspect to consider. The Shanghai Declaration offers a comprehensive framework for governments to fully harness the immense potential of health promotion. Health promotion is a collaborative endeavor that involves the integration of various principles, policies, and actions to ensure the well-being of all individuals. Embracing health promotion allows individuals to contribute to the creation of a healthier and more resilient world. This brings them closer to the goal of achieving "Health for All."

1.9. The Significance of Health Promotion in Disease Prevention

Preventive health has gained significant traction as individuals strive to enhance their overall well-being and make more informed decisions. There are several key reasons why health promotion plays a crucial role in preventing diseases.

1.9.1. Developing Community Programs and Effectively Communicating Health Information

Medical attendant professionals are often focused on providing direct patient care, as well as disease prevention. It is crucial to disseminate knowledge about diseases and the necessary precautions to safeguard patients, as this plays a vital role in preventing the spread of illnesses. Health practitioners have the opportunity to disseminate information to the community through educational sessions and individual counseling with their patients. This allows them to effectively communicate important knowledge in different formats. It is crucial for individuals to have a clear understanding of the potential risks that come with certain lifestyle choices in order to effectively initiate positive changes. One possible starting point could be to educate the general public about the importance of regular exercise (Winett, 1995).

Secondary prevention is another crucial aspect of health promotion. This primarily focuses on the vulnerability of individuals to specific illnesses and potential risk factors, rather than examining the collective characteristics of a community. Secondary prevention is a crucial aspect of healthcare that aims to minimize the transmission of diseases and assess the likelihood of infection when a patient receives a diagnosis from a healthcare professional. When residing in an area with elevated rates of obesity, drug and alcohol abuse, tobacco use, and poor nutrition, it becomes crucial to assist healthcare professionals in honing in on more targeted issues. This will greatly aid in the development of a prevention program tailored to a specific community.

1.9.2. Discussing the Dangers Associated with Alcohol Consumption, Smoking, and Drug Abuse

Research has established a clear connection between excessive alcohol consumption and an elevated risk of liver disease, high blood pressure, and stroke. Alcohol use can have a range of consequences, including risky behavior, social issues, job loss, strained relationships with family members, and difficulties learning and remembering (Winett, 1995). Despite the grave dangers of driving under the influence, there are individuals who (under the false assumption of their own capabilities) choose to operate a vehicle while heavily intoxicated. Health practitioners are well-equipped to educate patients and their families about the risks and symptoms associated with alcoholism. In addition, they can offer valuable resources and materials to help patients in their search for assistance. Smoking can lead to various health conditions such as emphysema, chronic obstructive pulmonary disease (COPD), lung cancer, and heart disease. According to the Centers for Disease Control and Prevention (CDC), individuals who smoke have a significantly higher risk of dying from COPD compared to those who do not smoke. The statistics show that smokers are 12 to 13 times more likely to succumb to this disease. It is important to note that smoking is a significant factor in almost 90% of lung cancer cases. Exposure to secondhand smoke has been associated with a range of health issues in infants and children, including ear infections, sudden infant death syndrome (SIDS), respiratory infections, and frequent severe asthma attacks.

Health practitioners play a crucial role in helping smokers quit by offering valuable support, sharing important information, and utilizing their expertise to develop and execute effective tobacco cessation programs. Drug abuse has a profound impact on both the mind and body of individuals. According to statistics, substance abuse is responsible for a higher number of illnesses, disabilities, and deaths compared to any other preventable health condition. Health issues such as nausea, vomiting, seizures, strokes, cardiovascular conditions, and weakened immune systems can arise as a consequence of drug abuse. Health practitioners possess the necessary knowledge and expertise to effectively recognize and address the symptoms associated with drug abuse. Through the provision of helpful next steps and the availability of materials and resources for treatment, patients and their families can be instilled with a sense of hope.

1.9.3. Encouraging the Importance of Regular Medical Examinations

Regular health assessments are vital components of health promotion and disease prevention, as stated by Winett, (1995). By conducting regular screenings, a primary care provider can carefully observe any changes in a patient's health, leveraging their established relationship to provide comprehensive care. It is highly advisable for individuals to schedule regular annual check-ups with their healthcare provider in order to minimize the risk of undetected health problems. When health practitioners are developing programs for prevention in their communities, it is important for them to consider raising the issue of free health screenings as part of their public outreach and educational programming. This can be a valuable way to engage with the community and promote preventive healthcare. Health insurance plans provide coverage for annual preventive checkups and vaccines, which in turn helps patients gain a better understanding of their rights and benefits. It is important to note that taking care of existing conditions is a crucial aspect of preventive care. This is because certain behaviors can either facilitate the management of diseases or alleviate symptoms. Regular counseling and support from health practitioners and other members of the care team can empower patients to take control of their health and lead more fulfilling lives.

1.9.4. Offering Assistance and Conducting Follow-Up

Individuals who are implementing substantial changes to their lifestyle in order to enhance their well-being and decrease their chances of developing illnesses often need continued support. Health practitioners have the ability to offer patients this follow-up method, serving as a valuable resource to enhance their likelihood of achieving positive health outcomes. It is crucial for individuals to have a strong support system to maintain healthy eating and physical activity habits. Without this support, there is a heightened risk of falling back into unhealthy patterns, which can lead to the development or worsening of diseases and health conditions. Health practitioners are expected to play a more proactive role in encouraging patients of all ages to improve their health. This is because health promotion and disease prevention, through adopting healthy lifestyles and making necessary changes, are becoming increasingly important in medical care. It is important to recognize that the responsibility for leading healthier lives lies with individuals. However, health practitioners play a crucial role in educating, informing, and supporting those who are ready to embark on a journey towards a healthier lifestyle.

1.10. Methods for Promoting Health

Participation in health promotion and illness prevention programs is beneficial for people of all ages. Health communication, health information, policy change, system change, and environmental factors are all possibilities for programs that aim to improve people's health and reduce the prevalence of disease.

1.10.1. Health Communication

According to a 2006 study by Jackson et al., health communication is the study and application of communication strategies with the goal of informing and influencing community and individual decisions that improve health. Health communication encompasses strategies that encourage and support individuals, communities, and groups to make healthier choices. Health communication often draws from multiple theories and models to promote beneficial changes in behavior and mindset. Health communication is connected to social marketing, which entails the development of programs and events aimed at influencing people to change their behavior for the better.

Jackson et al. (2006), list the following as effective components of health communication.

- Utilizing research-based strategies to shape products and materials and carefully selecting distribution channels for them. Having a deep understanding of conventional wisdom, ideas, terms, and priorities of different cultures and settings is crucial.
- Considering the health literacy of the audience, their internet access, exposure to media, and cultural competence. The materials cover a wide range of media outlets, such as social media posts, brochures, billboards, newspaper articles, radio commercials, television broadcasts, public service announcements, newsletters, videos, digital tools, case studies, group discussions, health fairs, field trips, and workbooks. Health messages can be effectively conveyed through different communication methods, including interpersonal interactions, small group discussions, community-level campaigns, and mass media platforms.

Health communication strategies have the potential to shape people's knowledge, attitudes, and behaviors.

- One way to achieve this is by increasing individuals' perception of risk, prompting them to take positive actions.
- It is important to conform to societal expectations and norms.

- It is important to ensure that necessary services and support are easily accessible to everyone.
- Empower individuals to make positive changes to their health and well-being.

When crafting health communication or social marketing strategies, it is crucial to consider the intervention's overarching communication goals. To make sure the content is relevant, you have to know who you're writing for. Messages must be customized according to the chosen method of communication. In addition, using a variety of communication and media strategies will guarantee wider reach. It is also crucial to make sure that the people you are trying to reach can hear you through the channels you are using.

1.10.2. Health Information

When individuals have access to opportunities to learn about health-related subjects, they are better equipped to make healthy lifestyle choices and maintain them. The intended recipients are considered while formulating health education strategies. People can learn about the advantages and disadvantages of different health topics, as well as how to change their own behavior (in a safe environment), through health education programs.

Here are some traits shared by health education strategies:

- Overseeing a local area 'needs assessment' to identify resources, requirements, limitations, and opportunities.
- Organizing a set of classes and other learning activities that will help people improve their skills, outlook, and knowledge.
- Making sure program staff are proficient through training, staying true to the program model, and developing content and materials that reflect the learning styles of the intended audience are all essential.
- Implementing programs with a curriculum and materials that are well-planned and integrated in a way that is convenient for participants.
- Encouraging participation from the target demographic. You can choose to educate individuals, groups, or entire populations about health.

1.10.3. Policy Change

Health promotion and disease prevention strategies can only be effective if there is a positive shift in policies, systems, and environments (PSE). Aiming to promote healthy behaviors, policies, systems, and environmental change strategies work to make healthy choices easily accessible in the community. Change strategies at PSE are developed with long-term viability in consideration. Health promotion and disease prevention programs can use policy shifts to accomplish their goals. Decisions regarding policies are made by stakeholder groups, organizations, and agencies. Some examples of policy approaches include lobbying for legislation, implementing fiscal measures, taxing, and overseeing regulations.

1.10.4. Systems Change

This refers to a significant departure from the previous approach to problem resolution. Systems change impacts the purpose, function, and connections of an organization by addressing its beliefs, policies, goals, relationships, and culture. Planned new procedures and interventions based on an established model of health promotion are one example of how the systems for promoting health and preventing disease are evolving.

1.10.5. Environmental Change

Changing the physical, social, or economic settings that influence health outcomes is one way to implement environmental change strategies. When addressing population health outcomes, environmental strategies work best when applied in tandem with other approaches. More parks, greenways, and trails in the community, along with signs encouraging people to walk and bike, are all ways to improve environmental health and reduce the likelihood of disease. Having more eateries, schools, and cafeterias provide nutritious, freshly prepared meals. This in one way or another helps in promoting health.

1.11. Challenges in Health Promotion

Before implementing health promotion and disease prevention programs, communities may need to tackle a few challenges, as highlighted by St Leger (2003). These challenges include:

- **Appropriate Communication Methods:** Utilizing various communication channels to engage with residents regarding the program can prove to be incredibly effective in terms of recruitment. To determine the most effective communication channels and gain insights into the preferences of the target audience, it is recommended to conduct focus groups, surveys, or other assessments to gather information on their information consumption habits.
- **Keeping the Community Motivated:** One crucial aspect of achieving success in program planning is the ability to keep the community motivated. Program planners must recognize that recruiting and retaining participants is a key factor in achieving this goal. Engage in educational initiatives and outreach programs to assess the level of community awareness regarding health issues, ascertain the expectations of community members, and inspire individuals to strive for improved health outcomes.
- **Cultural and Social Issues:** Unique cultural and social norms can have a significant impact on the program's chances of success. Communities often possess rich traditions and cultures related to food, alongside a tendency to be skeptical of medical professionals and outsiders, or to hold strong social beliefs regarding certain behaviors. It is important to actively acknowledge and comprehend these norms prior to implementing the program and devise strategies to effectively deal with them. Engaging individuals from the target population in this process can be instrumental in fostering cultural competency and promoting active involvement.
- **Resources and Sustainability:** Communities often face the challenge of limited financial, technological, and workforce resources when it comes to sustainability and resource management. It is important to note that program staff may have other activities and commitments to attend to. To establish long lasting support for the program, it is crucial to emphasize a common vision and actively engage partner

organizations and a broader group of community members.

- **Barriers to Participation:** Another factor that can affect the implementation and operations of a program is the local circumstances, such as geography. These circumstances can create barriers to participation. When designing the program, it is important to consider factors such as lengthy travel times, transportation availability (or lack thereof), childcare needs, and site availability. These considerations will help minimize any potential barriers that participants may face when trying to engage in the program.

1.12. Disparities in Public Health Data Access, Workforce Capacity, and Community Empowerment

Lee (2012) highlights the significant disparities in access to reliable public health data across different countries. It is crucial to establish strong information systems to effectively track progress towards health improvement objectives. When planning and evaluating health promotion programs, it is essential to incorporate readily available information as a standard practice. Furthermore, it is imperative to enhance the development and utilization of indicators that showcase the processes involved in health promotion and monitor the advancements made in promoting health, in order to not only decrease mortality and morbidity, but also to ensure continued progress. It is crucial to urgently incorporate information on health promotion, public health, and social determinants into globally comparable data systems.

There is a significant disparity among nations when it comes to the development of their workforce capacity and capability for health promotion. While some countries have made great strides in this area, others are lacking the necessary resources, or have none at all.

- It is imperative that there is a global push for increased investment in the education and training of health promotion specialists, practitioners, and other workers.
- It is crucial to include in essential training the evaluation of policies' impact on health and its determinants, the utilization of available information and evidence, the assessment of interventions, and the development of knowledge and skills for advocacy and mediation with politicians and the private sector.
- It is crucial to prioritize and continuously invest in enhancing the capacity for academic health promotion.
- It is important to recognize that health promotion is a separate field with its own unique knowledge base.
- It is also crucial to form partnerships with professionals and academics from related fields who have a common goal of promoting health (Lee, J. Y., 2012).
- It is crucial for disciplines such as public health, nursing, environmental health, education, psychology, the social sciences,

management sciences, development studies, and other related fields to establish robust connections and collaborations in order to enhance health promotion efforts.

- Professional accreditation programs play a crucial role in recognizing specialist competence in health promotion. By doing so, they contribute to the wider dissemination of knowledge and skills, as well as enhancing training and visibility in the field. In order to establish a clear framework and guide the development of educational programs, it is essential to reach a consensus on the fundamental skills and knowledge needed in the field of health promotion.

One of the fundamental principles of health promotion is to empower individuals and communities, recognizing and appreciating the valuable assets they contribute to improving health (Figure 1.4).

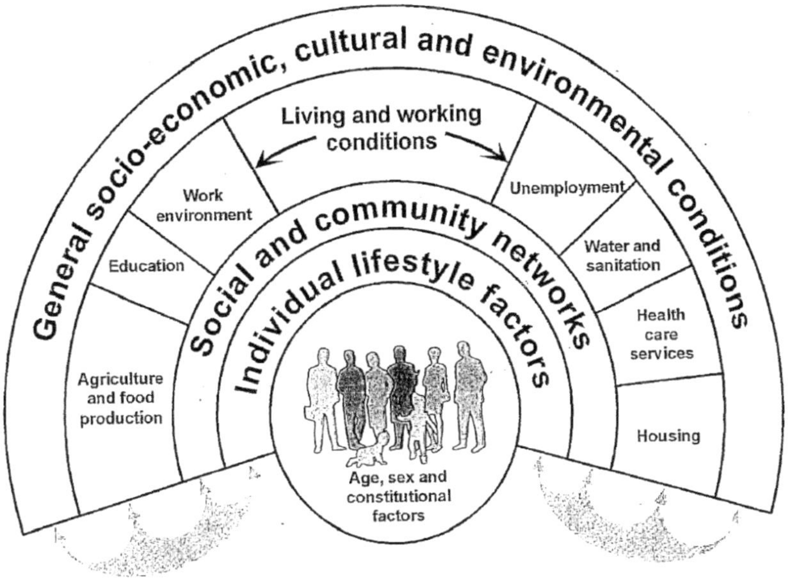

Figure 1.4. *Layers of influence on health.*

Source: Romeo-Velilla (2017).

Empowerment has proven to be a valuable tool in enhancing health and is widely recognized as a legitimate objective in the field of public health. Health promotion strategies that involve the community in program planning, policymaking, implementation, and evaluation have been proven to be effective and successful worldwide (Lee, 2012). The guiding principle for the widespread practice of including community voices in policy and planning processes is co-responsibility for action. Despite the lack of support from the national policy environment, health promotion has flourished at the community level. Effective health programs are best when they are seamlessly integrated into the daily lives of communities, aligning with local customs, and led by community members themselves. Civil society plays a crucial role in shaping policy at various levels, including local, national, and global, through advocacy, organizing, mobilization, consumer choices, and voting.

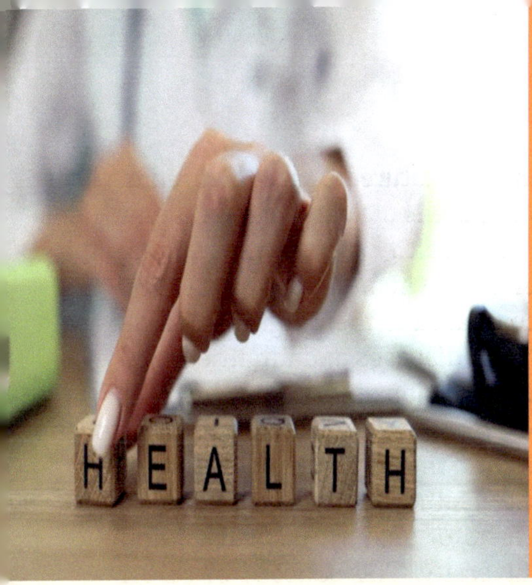

Chapter 2
DETERMINANTS OF HEALTH

Contents

2.1. Social Determinants

The conditions in which individuals are born, develop, and pass away are commonly referred to as social determinants of health (SDOH). The social determinants of health (SDOH) play a crucial role in shaping the knowledge, attitudes, beliefs, and behaviors of individuals and populations. For instance, they can influence lifestyle choices and behaviors, such as smoking, which in turn impact overall health and susceptibility to infections (Marmot & Wilkinson, 2005). Simultaneously, the general public has the ability to influence SDOH policy, thus potentially bringing about changes. It is crucial to grasp and address the significance of understanding and managing them as the field of social determinants of health continues to grow (Figure 2.1).

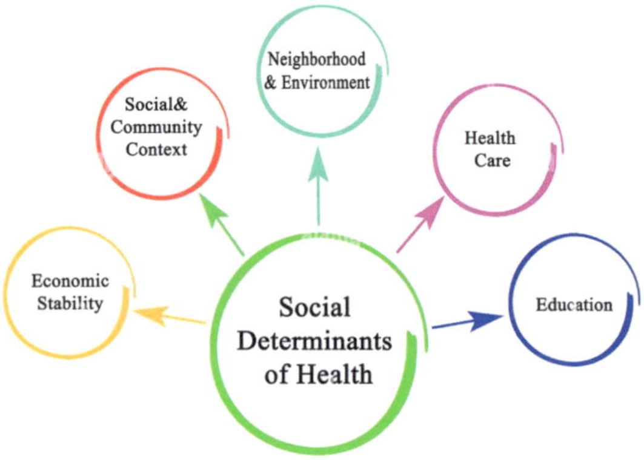

Figure 2.1. A chart showing the social determinants of health.

Source: Enitan (2022).

SDOH refers to the significant social structural influences on health and health systems. These influences encompass a wide range of factors, including social, physical, economic, and environmental aspects. It is important to recognize that these factors are shaped by government policies and have a direct impact on health. While the causal pathways may seem logical at first glance, it is important to consider the underlying concepts that influence them. The connections between these determinants and health are often complex and can involve multiple intervening factors. The complexity of this subject matter poses a significant difficulty when it comes to studying and ultimately addressing the important underlying factors. The social and economic factors that influence health play a crucial role in shaping individuals' well-being throughout their lives. Therefore, it is imperative that health strategies are closely linked to these factors. The longevity of health is influenced by unfortunate social and financial conditions. Individuals who find themselves lower on the social hierarchy often face a significantly higher risk of experiencing severe illness and premature death compared to those at the top. There is a clear social gradient when it comes to health, with lower-ranking office staff experiencing higher rates of infection and mortality compared to their higher-ranking counterparts. Many diseases and fatalities tend to be more prevalent among individuals in lower social strata (Marmot & Wilkinson, 2005). The material highlights the correlation between social status and health disparities, as well as the negative effects of anxiety, insecurity, and lack of social diversity. The concept of SDOH encompasses various structures and can be either relative or absolute in nature. Challenging circumstances can arise from various factors such as:

- Limited family assets
- Lower education levels during puberty
- Being stuck in a dead-end job or facing job insecurity
- Struggling with inadequate housing while raising a family

These obstacles often revolve around a specific demographic and their effects on health are intertwined. An important aspect of overall well-being is the reduction of educational setbacks, along with a strong emphasis on job stability and addressing income inequality within society. It is imperative to ensure that a reduced number of individuals experience falls, and that the distance of their falls is minimized. Housing and employment have a significant impact on education regulations and health standards. Strong societies are built on the foundation of providing all citizens with meaningful employment, financial security, and a sense of belonging. In contrast, areas where individuals experience insecurity, exclusion, and deprivation tend to be weaker and less resilient. Unemployment poses a significant threat to one's well-being, particularly in regions with high rates of joblessness. Research conducted in multiple countries has consistently demonstrated that unemployed individuals and their families face a significantly higher risk of premature death, even after accounting for various other factors. Unemployment is associated with various health consequences, including mental health issues and financial challenges, such as debt. It is evident that concerns about weakness can have a detrimental impact on one's overall well-being. Research conducted by Marmot & Wilkinson, (2005) has shown that there is a clear link between mental well-being and various health conditions such as anxiety, heart disease, self-reported illness, and depression, all of which are considered risk factors for coronary illness. Unsound or unstable positions can pose a risk, potentially resulting in adverse health effects. Contrary to popular belief, simply having a job does not guarantee the preservation of one's physical or psychological well-being. It is crucial to prioritize the quality of work. The economic transformations that occurred in the 1990s, along with the changes in work markets of industrialized nations, have led to a heightened sense of anxiety regarding job security. Job instability is a persistent stressor that becomes increasingly detrimental to one's health over time. It has been observed to have negative effects on both physical and mental well-being. Ultimately, addressing SDOH necessitates the implementation of a well-rounded strategy. Through the expansion of access to high-quality healthcare, education, and financial stability, as well as the establishment of robust social and physical conditions, we can promote health equity and overall well-being for everyone.

2.2. Economic Determinants of Health

Health economics encompasses a range of subjects, including resource allocation, healthcare system financing, and the impact of economic factors on health outcomes. It is a multidisciplinary field that explores these important areas. Having a grasp on the monetary factors that influence overall health is crucial for policymakers, healthcare providers, and researchers in order to develop effective strategies that promote the well-being of populations. This subtopic explores the significant correlation between financial aspects of healthcare and overall health, emphasizing the pivotal role of healthcare expenditure, access to medical services, health insurance, and economic factors. The impact of individual and societal healthcare expenditure on public health cannot be overstated. Higher medical care spending is often associated with improved medical services infrastructure, enhanced access to healthcare services, and improved health outcomes (Grossman, 2017).

Conversely, inadequate investment in healthcare can lead to subpar services, increased waiting periods, and limited availability of essential treatments. One of the challenges is finding the right equilibrium between providing top-notch healthcare and making efficient use of resources. The objective of health economics research is to identify healthcare delivery models and interventions that are cost-effective, ensuring that the available budgets are utilized efficiently and resulting in improved public health outcomes. Access to medical care is a crucial aspect of public health. The accessibility of healthcare is greatly impacted by various economic factors such as income, education, and location. Unequal access to healthcare often stems from socioeconomic inequalities, leading to disparities in health across different population groups. Efforts to enhance overall health should prioritize equitable access to healthcare services. This involves reducing barriers to access, expanding healthcare infrastructure in underserved areas, and ensuring that vulnerable populations have access to affordable and high-quality care. Health care coverage plays a crucial role in ensuring access to medical services and providing financial security. Individuals who have health insurance are more likely to benefit from preventive care, receive timely treatment, and avoid incurring high healthcare costs. Grossman (2017) argues that individuals without the protection of health insurance often encounter significant financial barriers to healthcare and may delay or forgo necessary medical services. Health financial specialists focus on analyzing the impact of various insurance models, such as private, public, and universal healthcare systems, on health outcomes and economic stability. Research findings provide valuable insights for policymakers seeking to enhance insurance coverage and enhance public health. Financial disparities are an inevitable concern when it comes to matters of healthcare finance. People with lower incomes and less education tend to experience poorer health outcomes, higher mortality rates, and limited access to healthcare services. These disparities are the result of the complex interplay between economic, social, and environmental factors. In order to effectively tackle health disparities, it is imperative to implement a comprehensive strategy that goes beyond the boundaries of the healthcare system. A comprehensive approach that tackles the underlying factors contributing to socioeconomic disparities, implementing policies aimed at alleviating poverty, enhancing education, and establishing social safety nets can yield substantial improvements in public health. Understanding health economics is crucial as it reveals the complex relationship between economic factors and public health outcomes. The health and well-being of populations are greatly impacted by factors such as healthcare expenditure, healthcare access, health insurance, and socioeconomic disparities. It is crucial for researchers and policymakers to recognize the importance of these economic factors and strive to develop policies and interventions based on solid evidence. These measures will not only improve public health outcomes but also ensure fair and equal access to healthcare. It is crucial to consider a comprehensive strategy that encompasses improvements to the healthcare system as well as broader social and economic policies in order to effectively address health disparities and enhance public health (Grossman, 2017). By striving for a more equitable healthcare system and tackling the root causes of health inequalities, we can make substantial strides in enhancing public health and providing everyone with the chance to live a healthier and more fulfilling life. Health economics remains a crucial factor in guiding these endeavors and attaining enhanced health outcomes for all individuals.

2.3. Environmental Determinants of Health

One of the major concerns in today's society is the detrimental impact of our modern lifestyle on the environment, which in turn leads to a rise in health hazards. Acid rain, ozone depletion, and various other global factors have a significant impact on human health. The hazards that have emerged due to these significant environmental disruptions are a direct consequence of human activity, presenting a serious threat to the survival of our species.

The survival, functioning, and growth of an organism are greatly impacted by various environmental factors. These factors encompass any observable component of the surrounding environment. Ecological variables encompass all factors that alter the natural environment. Certain components are visible, while others remain concealed. The ecological elements include air, water, environment, soil, normal vegetation, and landforms. The ecological elements play a crucial role in shaping health disparities across different geographic regions (Krause, Schaefer, & Highfield, 2021). The interaction between human and natural factors has a significant impact on human health, whether it be direct or indirect. There are five key environmental factors that play a significant role in shaping our surroundings:

2.3.1. Pollution

This is the act of introducing harmful substances, organic molecules, or pollutants into the Earth's atmosphere, water, or soil. This can be caused by natural events, such as forest fires, or by human activities, such as emissions from vehicles, factories, and nuclear waste. There are several types of pollution that we need to be aware of. These include air pollution, soil contamination, noise nuisance, water contamination, and radioactive contamination (Figure 2.2).

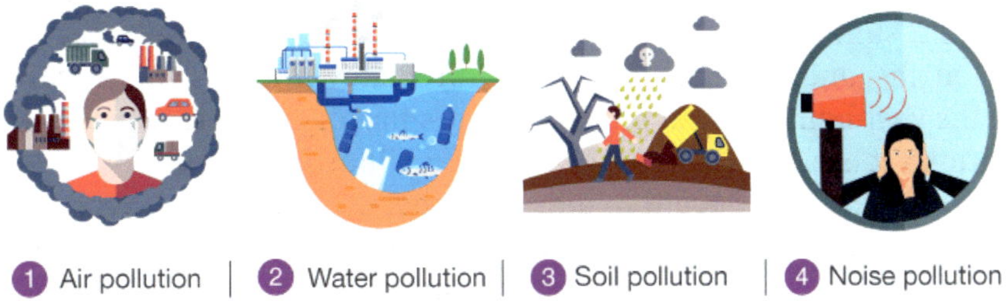

Figure 2.2. *Types of pollution chiefly arising as a result of anthropogenic causes.*

Source: Admin, 2022.

2.3.2. Deforestation

Deforestation refers to the process of tree removal. These can serve purposes related to human use and habitation, or they can occur naturally. Deforestation has a significant impact on the environment. One of the most significant issues affecting the environment is the lack of trees and forests. This deficiency not only contributes to climate change but also gives rise to a multitude of other ecological concerns.

2.3.3. Solid Waste

Solid waste pollution is another form of pollution that joins the ranks of air, water, noise, and soil pollution. Solid waste pollution occurs when various types of waste, including garbage, construction debris, metal fragments, glass and plastic products, decaying matter, agricultural waste, medical waste, and radioactive materials, are not properly disposed of.

2.3.4. Global Warming

Global warming is the phenomenon where the Earth's atmosphere and water bodies experience a gradual increase in average temperature. This natural issue is primarily caused by the increased levels of ozone depleting substances, such as carbon dioxide and methane, which are released through the burning of fossil fuels, emissions from vehicles, industries, and other human activities.

2.3.5. Shift in Climatic Conditions

Climate change is the result of various factors. The climate is significantly affected by global warming and the increasing concentration of greenhouse gases in the atmosphere. Climate change is having a detrimental impact on the environment. These encompass the physical, chemical, and biological characteristics of environments. Humans play a significant role in contributing to climate change, alongside natural disasters (Krause, Schaefer, & Highfield, 2021). Natural variables play an active role in shaping our health rather than simply being passive consumers. In order to achieve prosperity, it is crucial to have clean air, a stable environment, sufficient water, proper sterilization, safe lodging, and strong networks. Indeed, to ensure the well-being of both present and future generations, it is crucial that we give utmost importance to policies, education, and collective action when striving for healthier environments.

2.4. Behavioral Determinants of Health

An intricate interplay between behavior and health outcomes greatly influences an individual's well-being. Behavioral determinants are of utmost importance in assessing health conditions within a population. Behavioral determinants encompass various aspects of our lives, such as lifestyle choices, routines, and everyday actions. The ways in which individuals behave have a profound impact on their health outcomes. These behaviors can have both defensive and adverse effects (Agnikula, Singh, & Joy, 2021).

Understanding the significance of choices is crucial as they can greatly influence an individual's overall well-being. Diets, in particular, play a pivotal role in determining one's health. Eating a well-balanced diet that includes lean proteins, whole grains, fruits, and vegetables is essential for improving overall well-being. Excessive consumption of processed foods, sugary beverages, and high-fat meals can lead to obesity, diabetes, and cardiovascular disease. It is crucial to recognize the importance of everyday tasks. Engaging in regular practice has numerous benefits for our overall well-being. It positively impacts cardiovascular health, strengthens our muscles, and enhances our mental well-being. Living a sedentary life (where we don't engage in enough physical activity) can increase the likelihood of developing conditions such as obesity, osteoporosis, and depression. Smoking plays a significant role in influencing behavior. Smoking leads to cellular breakdown in the lungs, coronary illness, and respiratory problems. It is important to note that individuals who do not smoke can also experience negative health effects when they are exposed to secondhand smoke. When it comes to beverage consumption, it is crucial to practice moderation and responsible alcohol consumption. Excessive drinking leads to a range of negative outcomes, including addiction, accidents, and liver diseases. In the realm of social dynamics, one cannot underestimate the influence of social standards and the impact of friends when it comes to alcohol consumption. For example, using medication in an unauthorized manner can pose significant risks to both the body and mind. It is widely recognized that the consumption of illicit drugs has detrimental effects on an individual's overall well-being and physical condition. Drug use is strongly associated with addiction, overdose, and the transmission of infectious diseases such as HIV. Education, programs for reducing harm, and rehabilitation play a vital role in addressing societal challenges.

2.4.1. The Impact of Health Behavioral Determinants on Equity in Health

The "social gradient" is a consistent pattern that is often observed in populations. According to the social gradient, the availability of nutritious choices is impacted by one's socioeconomic status (Agnikula, Singh, & Joy, 2021). Structural barriers pose significant challenges for vulnerable populations when it comes to adopting healthy behaviors. Health education plays a crucial role in empowering individuals to make informed choices by providing them with knowledge about healthy behaviors. Positive behaviors are fostered through the implementation of supportive environments, such as the establishment of bike lanes and smoke-free zones. Ultimately, the course of our health is shaped by our behaviors, which should not be viewed as isolated incidents. It is within the power of every individual to contribute to the development of healthier communities. By cultivating a culture of well-being, overcoming obstacles, and encouraging healthy choices, we can all play a part in this collective effort.

2.5. Cultural Determinants of Health

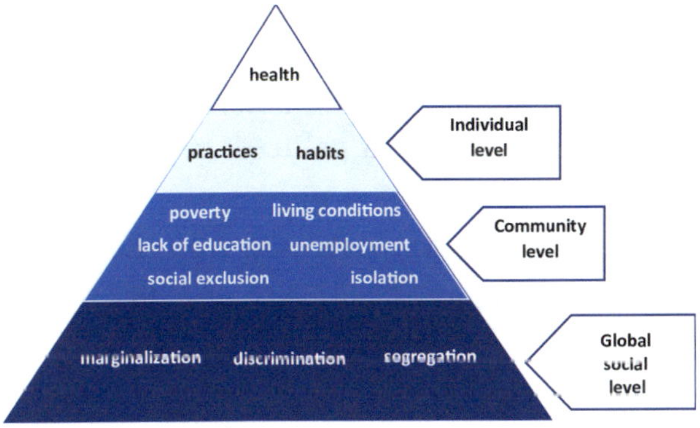

Figure 2.3. *Baseline model of social and cultural determinants of the health.*

Source: Milas & Klarić (2022).

Culture encompasses a collection of ideas, practices, and norms that are commonly embraced by a specific group of individuals or society. These patterns serve to distinguish members from those belonging to other groups and to identify them as members of a specific group. Considering the multitude of factors that can influence a culture, it is common to find a great deal of diversity within any given social group (Dressler & Oths, 1997). It can be beneficial to summarize clear characteristics of a particular culture, but it is important to avoid oversimplification (Figure 2.3).

According to Dressler and Oths (1997), culture encompasses a wide range of factors including ethnicity, language, religion, gender, financial class, age, sexuality, location of origin, upbringing, and educational experience.

Culture possesses several key characteristics. Firstly, it is constantly evolving and dynamic, adapting to the changing times. Secondly, it is a learned behavior that has been passed down through generations. Additionally, culture is often divided among individuals who have different perspectives on how they define and embrace reality. It is frequently recognized symbolically, expressed through language, dress, music, and behavior, and it becomes an integral part of a person's life.

2.5.1. The Impact of Culture on Health

Health is a concept deeply influenced by culture, as it molds individuals' perspectives and experiences of the world. Culture plays a significant role in defining various factors related to health and illness. The beliefs surrounding health and the cause of diseases among patients and medical professionals can be markedly influenced by cultural. As an example, it is worth noting that certain patients may lack knowledge about the germ theory and instead adhere to beliefs such as fatalism, the concept of the "evil eye," or the existence of a demon or djinn (a malevolent spirit in rural Afghanistan believed to cause illnesses resembling tetanus in infants). Some individuals may refuse to accept a diagnosis and maintain the belief that they have no control over the outcome. Instead, individuals must come to terms with the current state of affairs. Depression is often stigmatized in various cultures, where seeking help from a psychiatrist can unfortunately carry negative connotations. In certain societies, the perception of being "solid" (or what Canadians would consider "overweight") is associated with having a reserve of energy to guard against starvation. Interestingly, in these societies, "solid" women are often considered attractive and healthy.

Understanding the ways in which individuals perceive and communicate their experiences of illness and pain. In certain cultures, it is common for individuals to display stoicism even when experiencing intense pain. Conversely, in others cultures, individuals openly communicate emotions that may be considered somewhat distressing. Consequently, there can be differences in the extent to which pain needs to be examined or addressed.

It is crucial to take into account the location, method, and potentially the timing of a patient's search for help. Some societies tend to advise seeking care from allied healthcare providers initially, reserving a visit to the doctor for more severe issues. Across various cultures, it is considered a sign of respect to refrain from making direct eye contact. However, a caregiver who is unfamiliar with this norm may question whether this behavior indicates depression in their patient. Thus, it is important to consider the level of understanding and consistency with treatment choices suggested by medical care providers who may have different social beliefs. Some patients believe that a doctor who refrains from administering an injection may not be taking their symptoms seriously. Some patients also believe that any clinical service without the use of intravenous fluids (I.V. fluids) is incomplete.

Health is influenced by culture in various ways, as pointed out by Dressler and Oths (1997). One such way is through the acceptance of a diagnosis, which involves considerations such as who should disclose it, when it should be disclosed, and how it should be disclosed.

- Recognition of preventive or health advancement measures is crucial in maintaining overall well-being. These measures include vaccinations, prenatal care, contraception, and screening tests, among others.
- An important factor to consider is how individuals perceive their level of control when it comes to disease prevention and management.
- Perspectives on death, mortality, and the individuals that should be included.
- When it comes to communication, one important consideration is deciding between direct and indirect methods.
- Eye contact can be interpreted differently based on cultural norms. It is important to consider these differences when determining what is considered polite or rude.
- It is important to be prepared to discuss any potential side effects with your healthcare provider or use a mediator if necessary.
- Family dynamics encompass various aspects, including traditional gender roles, filial responsibilities, and patterns of family support.

2.6. Genetic Determinants of Health

The genetic makeup of DNA plays a crucial role in determining an individual's health and susceptibility to different conditions. These hereditary determinants play a crucial role in influencing biological processes, the likelihood of developing diseases, and overall well-being.

Genetics, as defined by Martin, Bergman, and Barzilai, (2007), involves the inheritance of genes from both sets of parents. Genes play a crucial role in shaping our physical characteristics (e.g., eye color).

Genetic predisposition is characterized by an elevated probability of developing a disease due to an individual's genetic composition. This outcome is a result of specific genetic variations that are typically passed down from a parent. Genetic predisposition plays a significant role in determining the likelihood of the disease occurring, although it is not the sole cause.

There are various genetic disorders that one may come across. Some examples of these disorders are:

- **Cystic Fibrosis:** This is a genetic disorder that affects the lungs and other organs. It is caused by a mutation in the CFTR gene, which leads to the production of thick, sticky mucus in the body. This mucus can clog the airways and make it difficult to breathe.
- **Brittle Bone Disease:** Also known as *Osteogenesis Imperfecta*, this is a genetic disorder characterized by fragile bones that are prone to fractures. This condition affects the body's ability to produce collagen, a protein that provides strength and flexibility to the bones. Individuals with Brittle Bone Disease often experience frequent fractures, even from minor trauma or normal.
- **Phenylketonuria (PKU):** This is a metabolic disorder that affects the body's ability to process an amino acid called phenylalanine.
- **Huntington's Disease:** This is a neurodegenerative disorder that affects the brain. It is characterized by the progressive loss of motor control, cognitive decline, and psychiatric symptoms. The disease is caused by a mutation in the huntingtin gene, which leads to the production of a toxic protein that damages nerve cells.
- **Kleinfelter Syndrome:** This is a chromosomal disorder that affects males. It is caused by the presence of an extra X chromosome, resulting in a total of 47 chromosomes instead of the usual 46. This condition can have various physical and developmental effects on individuals. Some common symptoms include:
  - A more elongated physique with reduced muscle mass
  - Increased hip width and elongated limbs
  - Enlarged breasts (a medical condition known as gynecomastia)
  - Decreased bone strength
  - Decreased energy levels
  - Reduced size of the penis and testicles
  - Delayed or incomplete puberty (also known as pubertal delay or hypogonadism)
- **Down's Syndrome:** This is a genetic disorder caused by the presence of an extra chromosome. It is characterized by certain physical features and intellectual disabilities.

Disease is seldom caused by a single gene or even multiple genes. On the contrary, most illnesses are complex and arise from the interplay between genetic factors and environmental influences. Environmental factors encompass a wide range of elements, including chemicals in the air or water, pesticides, diet choices, and household toxins. However, it is important to note that a family history of common diseases often plays a significant role in determining risk factors. Individuals with a family history of diseases such as cancer, diabetes, atherosclerosis, cardiovascular disease (CVD), autoimmune disorders, and mental illness have a higher likelihood of developing these conditions (Martin, Bergman, & Barzilai, 2007). Family members play a crucial role in understanding an individual's disease risk due to their close representation of the person's genomic and environmental interactions. Genetic variation that is inherited within families has a significant impact on the development of diseases, both in direct and indirect ways. One interesting aspect to consider is the occurrence of diseases at an earlier age than expected, sometimes even a decade or two before the general population typically develops them. Additionally, diseases that impact several close relatives can also be significant indicators of increased risk.

It is important to allocate some time to engage in meaningful conversations with your family. If possible, please review the death certificates and medical records of the family. It is important to gather information about your family members, including your grandparents, parents, siblings, aunts, uncles, nieces, and nephews. Search for data on major medical conditions and causes of death, including the period of illness, age at death, and ethnic background. People who come from families with a history of illness and who may have a genetic predisposition to certain diseases can greatly benefit from making lifestyle changes and undergoing regular screening tests. Family history revealing a consistent pattern of disease may suggest an inherited form of illness. Hereditary testing can be a valuable tool in determining the potential risk for relatives. One way to reduce the risk factors of type 2 diabetes is by adopting a healthy lifestyle. This includes maintaining a nutritious diet, engaging in regular physical activity, prioritizing sufficient sleep, and undergoing appropriate medical screenings. Lifestyle medication is an effective approach to addressing and treating various noncommunicable diseases – the leading causes of increased morbidity and mortality worldwide (Martin, Bergman, & Barzilai, 2007).

By examining the health conditions that run in our families, we can gain insights into our own potential risks and take proactive steps to prevent or manage them. This knowledge allows us to make informed decisions about our lifestyle choices, such as diet and exercise, and to seek appropriate medical screenings and interventions. By harnessing the power of family health history, we can empower ourselves to prioritize our well-being and make choices that promote long-term health. Early onset health issues can potentially signal a heightened familial risk. It is important to note that while genes are not mutable, one has the ability to modify their behavior. Understanding the health history of one's family is crucial for identifying potential risks associated with shared genes. If at all possible, attempt to gain a deeper understanding of the lifestyle and environmental factors that your family has in common, and understand the connection between adopting healthy lifestyles and reducing the likelihood of developing illnesses.

It is important for individuals to engage in open and honest conversations about their health with their family members; it is equally important for individuals to inform their medical care provider about any hereditary illnesses within their family. Children receive pairs of genes from their parents. When a child is conceived, they inherit one set of genes from their father and another set from their mother. Genes have the remarkable ability to come together in a multitude of ways, resulting in a vast array of unique combinations. This is the reason why certain family members bear a striking resemblance to one another, while others exhibit no physical similarities whatsoever. It is worth noting that genes can play a significant role in determining the likelihood of certain health conditions within a family. In addition to that, families also tend to have similar habits, diet, and environment. These factors play a crucial role in determining an individual's long-term health. It is important to note that individuals often share various aspects of their lives with their family members, including factors that may contribute to their health conditions. Some diseases are caused by a change in gene instructions – a phenomenon commonly referred to as a mutation. It is important to note that there are a multitude of mutations present in every individual. There are instances where these progressions have little to no impact or may even be slightly advantageous. Nevertheless, it is important to note that they can sometimes transmit illnesses. Common illnesses typically arise from a combination of factors, including changes in one's body, lifestyle choices, and current environment. It is also worth noting that individuals with similar genetic makeup may still be susceptible to different diseases based on their lifestyle choices or the environment they live in. Many illnesses can be attributed to a specific alteration in the DNA of a single gene. Several of these illnesses are not frequently encountered. These circumstances typically arise when a person is born with a mutated gene.

2.7. Access to Healthcare

Having access to medical care services is crucial for maintaining good health. However, certain communities encounter various obstacles when it comes to accessing these services. The concept of access to healthcare revolves around the timely utilization of personal health services to attain optimal health outcomes (Baeten et al., 2018). Ideally, individuals should have the ability to easily and confidently access a range of services, including primary care, dental checkups, social health, emergency care, and general health services (Figure 2.4).

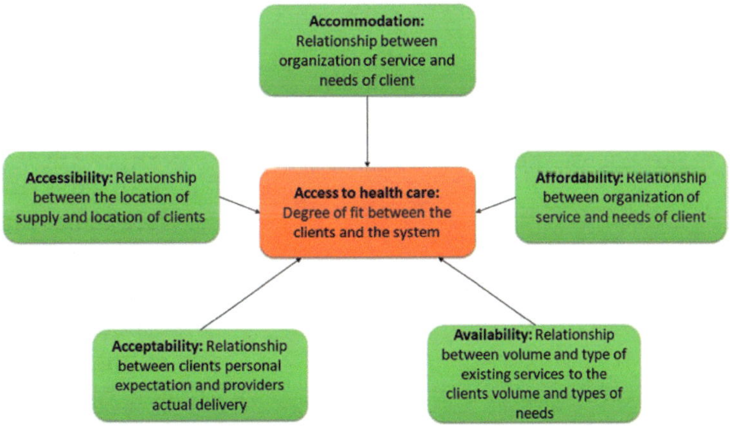

Figure 2.4. *The multi-dimensional concept of health care access.*

Source: Ouma et al. (2021).

Healthcare accessibility plays a vital role in:

- Maintaining overall physical, social, and mental well-being
- Preventing sickness

- Treatment, diagnosis, and disease detection
- Finding personal satisfaction in healthcare
- Preventing unnecessary loss of life
- Life expectancy

Many individuals, particularly those living in rural areas, often face obstacles when it comes to accessing medical services, which can greatly impact their ability to receive the care they require. Access to medical care implies that individuals can readily and promptly obtain necessary medical services. There are additional factors that can pose challenges to accessing healthcare, even when the community has an ample supply of services. In order to ensure access to medical care, rural residents need to have certain resources. These include:

- Financial means, such as health or dental insurance that is accepted by healthcare providers to cover the cost of services.
- They also need the means to reach and utilize these services, such as transportation to medical facilities that may be located far away.
- They need the ability to take time off work to make use of these services.
- Having confidence in one's ability to communicate with healthcare providers, particularly when the patient is not fluent in English or has limited health literacy – circumstances that can also hinder efficient and effective access to healthcare.

One of the key issues in healthcare is the limited access that many people face (Baeten et al., 2018). This is a significant challenge that needs to be addressed to ensure that everyone has the means and opportunity to receive the care they need. The section below describes these factors in further detail.

1. **Lack of Available Transportation:** It is often necessary for rural residents to travel long distances to access medical care facilities, particularly for specialized services. This can have a significant impact on travel time, expenses, time spent away from work, and delays in receiving treatment in a timely manner. Furthermore, a lack of dependable transportation poses a significant obstacle to one's mental well-being. In urban areas, public transportation is generally available for patients to reach medical appointments. However, transportation services in rural areas often fall short. In rural communities, it is often observed that there is a larger percentage of elderly individuals who have chronic conditions requiring them to make multiple visits to outpatient facilities. This situation poses a challenge due to the lack of available public or private transportation options.
2. **Workforce Shortages:** The shortage of healthcare workers has a significant impact on the accessibility of medical services in rural areas. One important factor in ensuring access to medical services is having a reliable source of care, which relies on having an adequate healthcare workforce. According to some healthcare researchers, simply estimating supplier accessibility is not enough to fully understand medical services access. Examining the rates of nonuse, such as considering rural residents who struggle to find a suitable healthcare provider, can provide a more comprehensive understanding of the availability of a sufficient healthcare workforce for rural populations.

3. **Poor Health Literacy:** Health education can also serve as a barrier to accessing medical services. The ability to comprehend health information and instructions from healthcare providers is impacted by an individual's level of health literacy. This issue can be quite concerning in rural networks, where residents often face lower levels of education and higher rates of poverty. Having a low level of health proficiency can cause individuals to feel hesitant about seeking medical care. This hesitation may stem from fear or dissatisfaction associated with communicating with a healthcare professional. Furthermore, navigating the intricacies of the medical services framework can prove challenging for individuals lacking health proficiency skills.
4. **Social Stigma and Privacy Issues:** In rural areas, healthcare access can be hindered by social stigma and privacy concerns, which are exacerbated by the absence of anonymity. Rural residents may hesitate to seek treatment for mental health, substance use, sexual health, pregnancy, or common chronic illnesses due to unease or privacy concerns. Patients' sentiments can be influenced by their personal connections with their healthcare provider or other staff members in the healthcare facility. Patients may experience feelings of anxiety or concern about various individuals, often friends, family members, or colleagues, who may witness them seeking services for conditions that are typically not openly discussed, such as counseling or HIV testing services. One potential solution to address patients' concerns is to co-locate or integrate behavioral health and primary care services in the same building. This approach can help alleviate some of the challenges faced by patients and provide them with more comprehensive care.

There are several advantages to having access to primary care:

- Provision of preventive services, which play a crucial role in early disease detection
- Care coordination
- Lower all-cause, cancer, and heart disease mortality rates
- Reduction in low birth weight
- Improved health behaviors
- Improved overall health
- Lower healthcare costs

2.8. Health Disparities

Health disparities refer to variations in health status when compared to the overall population (Braveman, 2006). There are several common indicators that can help us understand the health disparities in certain populations. These indicators include:

- A higher rate of disease or disability
- A shorter life expectancy
- Higher rates of chronic pain
- A higher rate of death

In rural areas, several factors contribute to health disparities. These include geographic isolation, lower socioeconomic status, higher rates of health risk behaviors, limited access to healthcare specialists and subspecialists, and a lack of job opportunities. These factors all play a role in creating disparities in health outcomes. Rural residents are also less likely to have access to job-based health insurance coverage, and if they are low-income, they often do not qualify for public health insurance programs. Foundations, federal and state agencies, and membership organizations are working together to reduce disparities and improve health and overall well-being. Several organizations provide funding, information, and technical support to be utilized at the state, regional, and local levels. Additionally, there are organizations that collaborate with policymakers to enhance their understanding of the issues impacting population health and healthcare.

2.8.1. Factors That Contribute to Health Disparities

Health disparities have multiple causes that vary by region. Various factors have been identified as contributors to health disparities among individuals. These include access to healthcare and public health services, socioeconomic status, health-related behaviors, and chronic conditions. Additionally, geographical distance, infrastructure limitations, and provider shortages have also been recognized as significant factors.

- **Transportation:** The situation becomes even more challenging for rural patients who require specialized care and must travel long distances to receive it. Rural communities face limited access to general health services, as public health agencies in these areas operate with inadequate funding, neglected innovation needs, and limited physical and human resources. Additionally, reliable transportation can pose a significant obstacle for rural residents seeking medical care and general health services due to long distances, poor road conditions, and limited availability of public transportation options in rural areas.
- **Socioeconomic Factors:** Financial status and related factors are considered as part of the social determinants of health (SDOH). The social determinants of health encompass the various circumstances and conditions in which individuals are born, live, learn, work, play, love, and age. These factors have a significant impact on a wide range of health outcomes and risks, as well as overall well-being and quality of life. Social determinants of health encompass a wide range of factors that have a significant impact on our well-being. These include income and poverty, housing conditions, educational attainment, race/ethnicity, access to healthcare, health literacy, environmental health, and various other influences on our overall health and wellness.
- **Insurance Coverage:** Based on the research conducted by Braveman, in 2006, it was found that 58.5% of adults living in rural areas had private insurance coverage in 2020. In contrast, 43.5% of rural children had private insurance coverage. On the other hand, 26.3% of rural adults and 52.0% of rural children had public coverage. It was also observed that 17.9% of rural adults and 7.7% of rural children were uninsured. In comparison to populations in small, medium, large (fringe), and large (central) metropolitan areas, individuals living in rural areas had the lowest rate of private insurance coverage, the highest rates of public coverage, and the highest uninsured status.
- **Health Behaviors:** At the

community level, the adoption of positive health behaviors can significantly influence the rates of disparities in health status and mortality. Some common behaviors to consider are smoking, alcohol consumption, body weight management, and sexual behavior. The health of individuals varies based on their behaviors. Take into consideration that individuals who engage in sexual activities with multiple partners have a higher risk of contracting sexually transmitted infections in comparison to those who have only one partner or none at all.

- **Education Level:** Disparities in schooling are closely linked to variations in wellbeing. Leaving school is associated with a range of social and well-being issues. In general, individuals with lower levels of education are more likely to face a range of health risks, such as obesity, substance abuse, and intentional or accidental injuries, when compared to those with higher levels of education. Higher levels of education are associated with increased life expectancy and a greater likelihood of accessing and comprehending essential health information and services necessary for making informed health decisions. It has been found that there is a strong correlation between good health and academic success (Braveman, 2006). There is a strong correlation between higher academic grades among high school students and the adoption of more significant levels of defensive wellbeing behaviors, as well as lower levels of wellbeing risk behaviors.

2.9. Addressing Determinants Through Health Promotion

The health care delivery system is now taking into account the influential role of non-medical, social determinants of health. There is also a growing movement to include health impact/ outcome considerations in non-health policy areas (Schulz, Krieger, & Galea, 2002). These include various government and state initiatives, public health insurance initiatives led by states or health plans, and provider-level activities focused on identifying and addressing the non-clinical, social needs of their patients.

Government and state initiatives play a crucial role in shaping the policies and programs that impact our society. These initiatives are carefully designed and implemented to address the needs and challenges of our communities. Through strategic planning and collaboration, government and state initiatives aim to improve the quality of life for all citizens. By investing in various sectors such as education, healthcare, and infrastructure, these initiatives strive to create (Schulz, Krieger, & Galea, 2002)

In 2016, the Center for Medicare and Medicaid Innovation (CMMI), established under the Affordable Care Act, introduced a new model called the "Responsible Health Communities" model. This model aims to connect individuals enrolled in Medicare and Medicaid with community services to address their social needs related to health. The model provides funding to examine the impact of intentionally identifying and addressing the healthcare needs of federal medical insurance and Medicaid recipients through screening, referral, and community navigation services in relation to healthcare costs and utilization. In 2017, a total of 32 awards were granted by CMMI to associations for their participation in the model over a period of five years (Schulz, Krieger, & Galea, 2002). 12 recipients have been selected to provide route services, assisting high-risk individuals in accessing community services. Additionally, 20 recipients will work on partner coordination to ensure that community services are accessible and responsive to the needs of those enrolled.

The CMMI State Development Models Drive (SIM) involves the participation of multiple states in implementing multi-payer delivery and payment reforms that prioritize population health and acknowledge the influence of social determinants. The CMMI initiative SIM provides financial and technical support for health care payment and service delivery models that are led by the state and involve multiple payers. These models have the goal of enhancing health system performance, improving care quality, and lowering costs. Up until now, the SIM drive has provided nearly $950 million in awards to more than half of the states to design and test innovative payment and delivery models. State governments must develop a comprehensive strategy to improve population health as part of the second round of SIM grant awards (Schulz, Krieger, & Galea, 2002). States that have received Cycle 2 awards are actively exploring various strategies to identify and prioritize population health needs. They are working to connect clinical, public health, and community-based resources, while also addressing the social determinants of health.

Within the Medicaid program, there are several initiatives focused on reforming delivery and payment methods, with a particular emphasis on the intersection of social needs and healthcare. States like Colorado and Oregon are currently implementing Medicaid payment and delivery models that prioritize the integration of physical, behavioral, and social services. These models also emphasize community engagement and collaboration through regional entities. Furthermore, these endeavors could potentially fall under the purview of Section 1115 Medicaid demonstration waivers (Schulz, Krieger, & Galea, 2002).

Every Coordinated Care Organization (CCO) in Oregon must establish a community advisory council and carry out a community health needs assessment. CCOs are compensated with a global payment for each enrollee, allowing them to offer a wide range of "health-related services" that go beyond the usual Medicaid benefits and can also address the social determinants of health. Based on initial observations, it appears that CCOs are actively engaging with community partners and taking steps to tackle the social determinants of health through a range of projects. A study conducted by the Oregon Health & Science University's Center for Health Systems Effectiveness and published in 2017 discovered that CCOs were linked to decreases in spending growth and enhancements in certain quality areas. Based on the evaluation, the majority of CCOs expressed their belief that health-related flexible services were effective in enhancing outcomes and decreasing costs.

In Colorado, the Local Cooperative Associations (RCCOs) play a crucial role in connecting individuals to community services. These RCCOs are compensated monthly for each enrollee and work closely with providers to ensure that people's specific needs are addressed through referral systems and designated programs. An analysis published in 2017 comparing Oregon's CCO program with Colorado's RCCO program revealed that Colorado's RCCO program achieved comparable reductions in expenditures and days of ongoing care (Schulz, Krieger, & Galea, 2002). Several other state Medicaid programs have implemented Accountable Care Organization (ACO) models. Models frequently incorporate population-based payments or total cost of care formulas, incentivizing providers to address the comprehensive needs of Medicaid beneficiaries, including the social determinants of health.

Medicaid funds can be utilized to provide a range of housing-related services, including referral, support, and case management. These services are designed to help individuals connect with and maintain stable housing. As an example, the Louisiana Department of Health worked together with the Louisiana Housing Authority to create a Permanent Supportive Housing (PSH) program. This program has two main goals: to prevent and decrease homelessness, and to avoid unnecessary institutionalization of individuals with disabilities. While it is not possible for states to utilize Medicaid funds for room and board expenses, it is worth noting that Medicaid funds can be allocated towards a range of housing options. Louisiana's Medicaid program provides coverage for a range of services related to pre-tenancy, move-in, and ongoing tenancy for Medicaid beneficiaries residing in permanent supportive housing. As stated by Schulz, Krieger, and Galea, (2002), Louisiana has maintained an impressive housing retention rate of 94% since the program started accommodating tenants in 2008. According to an initial analysis conducted on the PSH program, it was discovered that Medicaid acute care costs decreased by 24% after individuals were provided with housing. Based on initial analysis, noteworthy decreases in hospitalizations and ER utilization have been observed subsequent to the implementation of the PSH intervention.

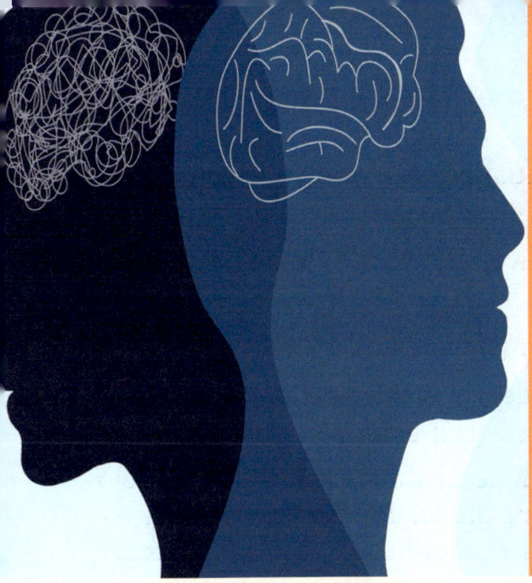

Chapter 3

MODELS OF HEALTH BEHAVIOR CHANGE

Contents

Janze and Becker, (1984) discuss the significant impact of the Health Belief Model, the Theory of Reasoned Action, and the Operant Learning Theory on the development of health education programs. Over the past decade, the Social Cognitive Theory (SCT) has gained significant recognition and has become the dominant model in the field of health education. Firstly, it is important to note that while the Health Belief Model and Theory of Reasoned Action primarily focus on cognition, it is worth highlighting that SCT goes beyond the study of knowledge and attitude. SCT also considers behavioral aspects such as social skills and the environment. In contrast to other theories that focus primarily on individual behavior, SCT takes a broader perspective by examining behavior at the group or collective level. SCT seeks to explain not only individual behavior, but also how individuals interact with the larger social system. Therefore, SCT could be considered a more suitable theoretical framework for the development of Comprehensive School Health Programs that include both individual and environmental factors. Given the prevalence of using SCT as a teaching method in health education, it is important to provide a concise overview of this model to demonstrate its usefulness for educators in this field.

3.1. Health Belief Model

The health belief model is a theoretical model that can be used to guide health promotion and disease prevention programs. This tool is used to analyze and predict individual changes in health behaviors. This particular model is widely utilized for understanding health behaviors (Figure 3.1).

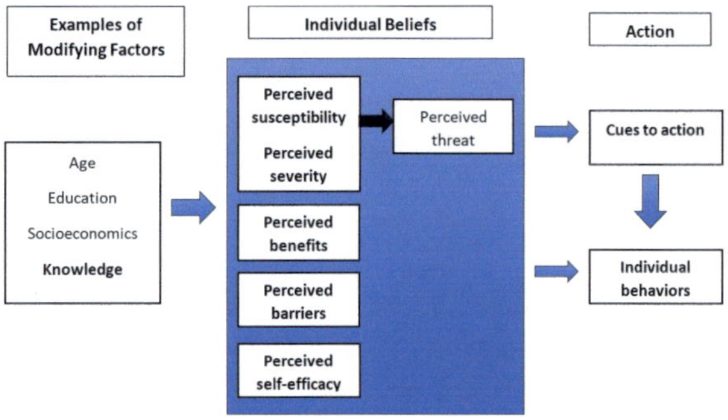

Figure 3.1. *Constructs of the health belief model.*

Source: Nelson et al. (2021).

The health belief model emphasizes the importance of personal beliefs regarding medical issues and how they influence individual health-related behaviors. The model outlines the crucial factors that influence a person's behavior in terms of their:

- Susceptibility to illness or disease (perceived vulnerability)
- Belief in the severity of the outcome (perceived seriousness)
- Potential benefits of taking action (perceived benefits)
- Perceived barriers to taking action
- Receptiveness to cues that prompt action (signals to activity)
- Confidence in their ability to succeed (self-efficacy)

One good example of the health belief model is the Michigan Model for Health. This is a comprehensive school-based curriculum that focuses on various important aspects of well-being, such as nutrition, physical activity, alcohol and drug use, safety, and personal health. It covers a wide range of topics that are relevant and relatable to students. This model modifies certain aspects of the health belief model related to information, skills, self-efficacy, and social support. Breast Cancer October is the designated month for Mindfulness Month – a yearly initiative aimed at raising awareness about breast cancer. This mission utilizes the health belief model to educate and inform the public (Janz & Becker, 1984). In the month of October, various organizations may provide complimentary screenings and educational programs to increase public awareness and detect early cases of breast cancer.

The Health Belief Model can assist in developing interventions, both in the short-term and long-term. The Health Belief Model's effectiveness in identifying crucial decision-making factors that impact health behaviors is determined by five essential action-related components. These components include:

- Gathering data through conducting a comprehensive needs assessment and employing various methodologies to determine the at-risk individuals and target populations
- Communicating the outcomes of risky behaviors in a straightforward

manner to determine their level of severity

- Emphasizing the benefits of following the suggested course of action and explaining the necessary steps
- Aiding in identifying and reducing barriers to action
- Demonstrating activities through exercises that promote expertise advancement and providing support to enhance self-adequacy and the likelihood of successful behavior changes

These activities cover important aspects of the health belief model and can be used to design or modify health promotion or disease prevention programs (Janz & Becke, 1984). The health belief model can be effectively utilized either on its own or in combination with other theories or models. In order to ensure a successful outcome with this model, it is crucial to identify the relevant and appropriate "prompts to activity" for the intended population.

3.2. Theory of Planned Behavior

Individual behavior is seen as a product of intentions in the theory of planned behavior. These intentions are predicted based on attitude, subjective norms, and perceived behavioral control (Figure 3.2).

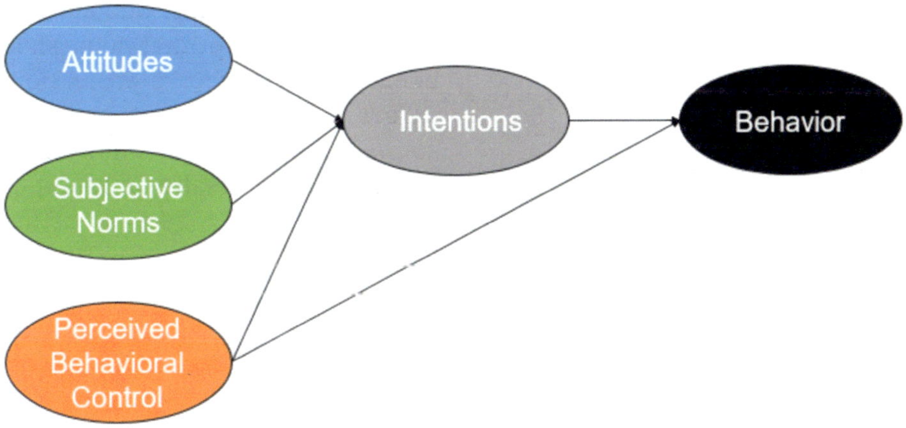

Figure 3.2. *The theory of planned behavior model.*

Source: Worthington, 2021.

Behaviors are influenced by intentions, which are determined by three factors: behavioral attitudes, behavioral norms, and perceived behavioral control. This is in line with the theory of planned behavior. According to studies, there is a possibility that an external factor can influence or restrict behavioral participation, regardless of an individual's intention. This is dependent on the level of control the individual has over their behavior and how well their perceived control aligns with their actual control.

For the case of introducing evidence-based instructional practices (EBIPs) as the desired behavior, factors related to teaching and learning in general, as well as factors specific to the use of EBIPs, are important in this context. Subjective norms can be seen as a form of social pressure, encompassing not only the individual's perception of what others expect them to do, but also their personal inclination to respond to this pressure. Each of the three groups would possess subjective norms. Students hold certain expectations regarding the teaching methods of STEM faculty, while colleagues and administrators have their own opinions on how they should teach (Ajzen, 1991). Self-efficacy refers to an individual's perception of their ability to successfully perform a behavior in a specific situation. It also includes self-efficacy in using EBIPs and the various external factors that can impact EBIPs, such as classroom environments, time constraints, and available resources. The likelihood of that action occurring increases as the three factors increase.

According to closely related theories, (i.e., the Theory of Reasoned Action and the Theory of Planned Behavior), an individual's health behavior is determined by their intention to engage in specific actions. The concept of behavioral intention, which holds great importance in this theory, elucidates that an individual's inclination to act in a particular manner is influenced by their attitude towards the behavior and their perception of social pressure associated with it. Subjective norms are influenced by the dynamics of groups and an individual's sense of control. Beliefs that are based on personal experiences and positive social norms can contribute to a stronger sense of control and a higher likelihood of translating intentions into actions.

A good example of a program that applies Theory of Reasoned Action/Planned Behavior is the SIPsmartER program. This is an initiative focused on preventing and controlling chronic diseases in the rural southwest Virginian setting. One of the main objectives is to decrease the intake of sugar-sweetened beverages among adults, as highlighted by Ajzen (1991). The selected intervention strategy is grounded in the Theory of Planned Behavior and encompasses educational methods such as small classes and teach-back approaches. The program was created to provide educational support to women residing in rural areas of Appalachian Kentucky, with the aim of raising awareness about cervical cancer prevention.

One approach to effectively addressing the program components is by enhancing knowledge, modifying attitudes, beliefs, and behaviors through the application of the Theory of Planned Behavior.

The theory of reasoned action/planned behavior is instrumental in understanding the factors that influence health behaviors and in guiding the development of health promotion and disease prevention programs. Subjective norms are a fascinating concept that helps shed light on the behavior of healthcare professionals, patients, carers, and various other members of the community. The application of these theories can be seen in health promotion and disease prevention efforts, such as asthma treatment compliance, smoking cessation programs, and campaigns against drug use.

There are assumptions and limitations of the Theory of Planned Behavior that must be considered. For instance, it suggests that individuals make rational decisions based on their attitudes, subjective norms, and perceived behavior control. Furthermore, it should be noted that these factors may not be actively considered during the decision-making process. Put simply, individuals may not explicitly express their opinions, yet these opinions can still have a significant impact on a specific choice.

One of the flawed assumptions of the rational choice theory is that individuals tend to make decisions driven by their emotions rather than rational thinking. According to certain researchers, it has been suggested that humans do not always behave or think in a rational manner, but rather, they can be described as "making sense".

3.3. Transtheoretical Model

The Transtheoretical model (TTM) is a widely recognized framework that has been extensively studied and applied in various fields. It provides a comprehensive understanding of behavior change and offers valuable insights into the stages and processes involved in making lasting changes. TTM has proven to be a valuable tool for researchers and practitioners alike, enabling them to better understand and address the complexities of human behavior. Hashemzadeh et al., (2019) have identified the stages of TTM as follows:

- Precontemplation
- Contemplation
- Preparation
- Action
- Maintenance

TTM has emerged as a widely utilized theoretical and clinical framework in the field of mental health. Its effectiveness has been demonstrated across a diverse range of areas, including smoking cessation, alcoholism treatment, weight control, exercise promotion, sun protection, prevention of sexually transmitted diseases, addressing bullying and school violence, managing addiction, promoting condom use, and encouraging preventive measures such as mammography and cancer screening (Figure 3.3).

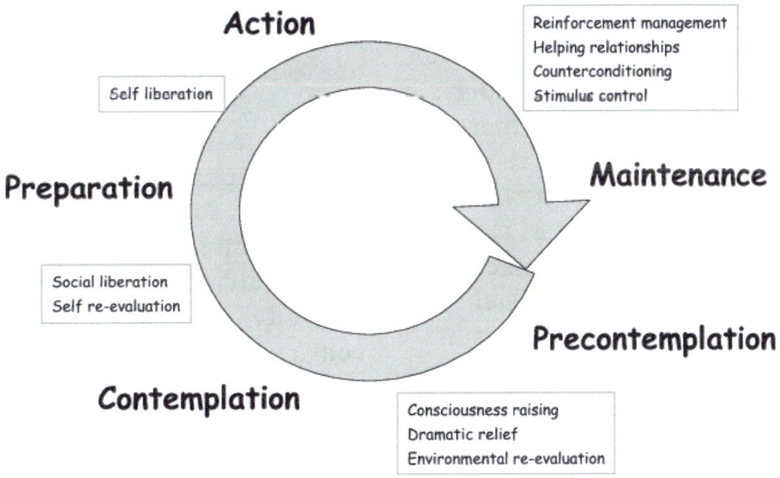

Figure 3.3. *The TTM of behavior change.*

Source: Adams (2004).

3.3.1. Pre-Contemplation

Most clients in this stage exhibit a lack of motivation and believe that there is no problem to be addressed. Consequently, they are not inclined to seek out a solution. Individuals at this particular stage may lack awareness or understanding of the issue at hand and may not fully grasp the consequences of their actions. This response is highly valuable as it differs from the majority of patients who tend to overlook their negative behaviors. This holds significant importance in the grief process as individuals find themselves in a state of denial, seeking to rationalize their actions. At this stage, individuals may exhibit an attitude of resistance, lack of motivation, and a reluctance to embrace change. In addition, these individuals tend to have a pessimistic outlook and focuses extensively on the potential negative consequences of change rather than highlighting the positive outcomes that could be achieved. When an individual who is not yet considering change seeks therapy, it is often due to the influence of those around them who have encouraged them to seek a solution. Under certain circumstances, individuals may exhibit certain traits when subjected to consistent and gradual pressure. Individuals in the precontemplation stage often do not proceed with positive changes as they no longer feel compelled to make those changes. The approach itself involves a form of therapy that aims to raise consciousness and can also be seen as a valid way to bring about changes in one's life situation. When individuals enter a new phase of life, they often take a moment to contemplate whether their actions are beneficial or detrimental to themselves and those around them. Even though someone may have come to this realization, they may still be in the initial stage of change because they haven't fully grasped this awareness.

3.3.2. Contemplation

This stage demonstrates a recognition of the behavior as being unacceptable, with a strong determination to eliminate it. However, there remains uncertainty regarding the necessity of addressing the problematic behavior. Consequently, these individuals will lack the motivation to engage in activities that can bring about change. Contemplation involves placing the "problem" or "context" at the forefront, with the actor/actress remaining stationary throughout. This is the point where individuals often find themselves caught in a state of uncertainty, grappling with conflicting thoughts and struggling to make a decision for an extended period of time. Typically, individuals at this stage are quite interested in learning about their behaviors and how to address any imbalances. Some people might respond by acknowledging that they have a problem and recognizing the need to take action. This form is commonly referred to as chronic contemplation or behaviorally procrastinating.

3.3.3. Preparation

During this phase of change management, individuals typically acknowledge the negative aspects of a behavior and express their determination to put an end to it. However, it is now widely acknowledged that the advantages outweigh the costs associated with changing one's behavior. People often seek out various sources of knowledge to address challenges and adapt to changes. They may turn to self-help literature, therapy, or change programs as they begin to plan their next steps. Gathering information is crucial for effective preparation. When individuals are excluded from the process, they often struggle to adequately plan or fully consider the impact of the impending change on themselves. Consequently, individuals may experience a highly precarious existence as they struggle to navigate through a multitude of challenges. This, in turn, significantly hampers their chances of achieving a successful recovery, as the likelihood of a relapse looms ominously. Proper organization is sometimes achieved when individuals sincerely commit to taking appropriate actions within a specific timeframe. Many people have already made significant progress in this regard over the past year. Individuals in this stage often express opinions such as, "smoking is an extremely unhealthy habit and the research I have been conducting provides compelling reasons for why one should attempt to quit smoking. Personally, I have been making efforts to reduce the number of cigarettes I consume".

3.3.4. Action

An important objective has been established to completely eliminate the negative behavior over the course of several months. During this stage, individuals begin to cultivate faith as they firmly believe in their own capacity and motivation to embrace further transformation. They emphasize the importance of the behavioral change and the level of dedication to oneself. At this point, individuals are prepared to embrace assistance and direction. Reinforcement of rewards is an effective method for providing short-term positive motivation. The emphasis here lies in recognizing potential challenges to recovery and developing effective strategies to minimize triggers that may lead to relapse. Behavioral changes at the highest level are not only recognized by the individual, but also by others. However, it is important to note that the changes in this stage should not be interpreted as the sole outcomes of the process. Many individuals tend to overlook the fact that implementing change requires careful consideration of the necessary preparations...instead focusing solely on the action itself. Engaging in such practice can lead to a dearth of comprehension and a sense of exasperation if the student embarks on this stage without adequate preparation. One might argue that individuals in the action stage often find it more convenient to vocalize their intention to quit smoking rather than taking concrete steps towards achieving their goal.

3.3.5. Maintenance

During the maintenance stage, the focus is on smoothly transitioning to the new behavior change. Within this category, the individuals have successfully abstained from engaging in any negative behavior for a period of over six months. At this stage, individuals develop a strong belief in the long-term effectiveness of their behavioral changes and experience a reduced sense of apprehension about reverting to old habits. One important aspect is the ability to proactively prevent new issues from arising. Additionally, it is crucial to maintain a comprehensive record of one's accomplishments. There might be certain circumstances that tempt individuals to revert to the past, but they are determined to resist this temptation to preserve the progress they have made through their transformations. The person has acquired the ability to anticipate circumstances that may result in a setback and devise strategies to overcome those situations and prevent a relapse. Typically, most people remain in this stage for a period ranging from six months to five years.

The primary objective of TTM is to develop a strategic course of action that enables individuals to effectively combat the risk of relapse and maintain a steadfast commitment to sobriety. It is important to address the concept of relapse and its connection to the process of change. At times, individuals may find themselves navigating through multiple stages before successfully adopting new behaviors. As an example, it is worth noting that individuals who smoke typically need to make three to four attempts before successfully maintaining long-term cessation. It is important for individuals to not view a setback in their success journey as a failure, particularly when taking into account the possibility of relapse. It is important to view this as a valuable chance to reassess the factors that prompt us to modify our behavior, the motivations behind our goal achievement, the assessment of obstacles that hinder our progress, and the development of more efficient action plans for unforeseen circumstances. It is important to recognize that there is always the possibility of relapse for this individual, and it should not be viewed as a negative occurrence.

Approximately 15 % of individuals experience a relapse, where they revert to the pre-contemplation stage and try to forget their previous attempts at change and the negative behavior itself. The majority of individuals (approximately 85%) tend to transition from the contemplation or preparation stage to another contemplation or preparation stage, rather than reverting back to the pre-contemplation stage. The treatment process for individuals involves regular intervention during the initial three to six months of abstinence. This time frame is critical as it is when individuals are most susceptible to relapse into substance use.

The final stage, known as the termination stage, often receives less attention in discussions about the stages of change. This is likely because reaching this stage can be quite challenging and demanding. It is a term used to describe a period when a client is not easily swayed and an individual has complete trust in the client (Hashemzadeh et al., 2019). Sometimes, achieving a high level of success can lead to certain addictive behaviors. However, similar patterns can be seen in our daily lives. For example, when we get into a car, we instinctively fasten our seat belts. Similarly, when we are reminded to take our medicine, we do so without thinking twice. In order to ensure the successful progression of the stages, it is imperative to have certain key elements in place. The theory encompasses several factors, such as the processes of change, decisional balance, and self-efficacy.

3.4. Social Cognitive Theory

The Social Cognitive Theory (SCT), originally known as the Social Learning Theory, was a significant development in the field of social psychology. It was formulated by Albert Bandura during the 1960s and began to emerge by 1986. SCT highlights the notion that learning is a collaborative process involving the individual, their environment, and their actions. This can be interpreted as a strong dedication to following guidelines that are rooted in the principles of social influence and the emphasis on both external and internal social reinforcements in SCT (Figure 3.4).

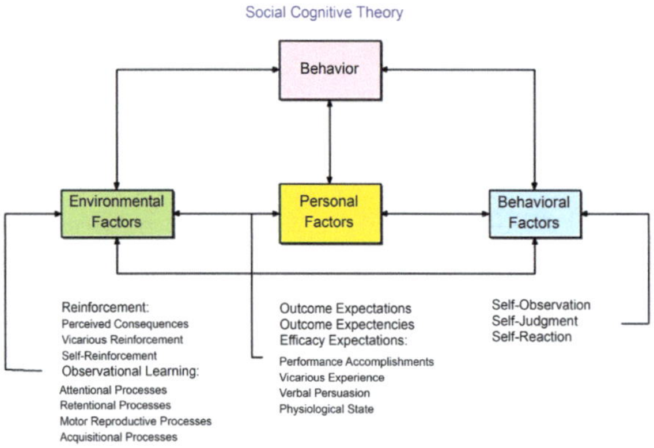

Figure 3.4. *Structural paths of influence articulated within social cognitive theory.*

Source: McCumber (2014).

One notable distinction of SCT is its focus on the process of individual learning and behavior, as well as the specific contexts in which these behaviors are displayed. Previous experiences play a significant role in shaping our behavior and the reasons behind it. They influence our expectations and the reinforcements that determine whether we will engage in a particular behavior.

Various theories of behavior are proposed for health promotion, but many of them overlook the importance of behavior maintenance. Consequently, they tend to prioritize the initiation stage. It is crucial to emphasize that the primary goal of public health is to sustain behavior rather than just initiating it. The objective of SCT is to analyze the ways in which individuals utilize control and reinforcement strategies to actively participate in desired behaviors that are self-directed and self-regulated.

As Social Learning Theory evolved into SCT (theories of self-efficacy and learning), the construct of self-efficacy was introduced along with the initial five constructs. As stated by Bussey and Bandura (1999), the constructs discussed in their research include attitudinal and behavioral competence. This concept pertains to an individual's fundamental capacity to engage in a behavior based on their knowledge and skills. Successful behavior can be analyzed from two main perspectives: its nature and its execution. Behavioral ethics plays a crucial role in guiding individuals to understand the impact of their actions and adapt to the world around them. Modeling suggests that individuals can observe and learn from others by watching their behavior and then imitating it. One way to showcase this concept is by observing and replicating certain behaviors. According to behaviorists, the ability to perform a task effectively can be acquired through observation of others who excel at ıt.

Consequences refer to the outcomes of a person's behavior, whether they are internal or external. These outcomes can either encourage or discourage someone from engaging in a particular behavior.

Reinforcements can originate from within the organism, driven by its own motivation, or they can come from external sources. These reinforcements can be either positive or negative in nature. This construct in SCT is highly comprehensive and intricately connected to the relationship between behavior and the contingency of the environment.

Anticipations are the expected results of one's actions. There are two potential sources of expectancy regarding our products: one related to health and the other unrelated to health. Humans have a tendency to plan ahead and consider the potential outcomes of their actions. They seek rewards or anticipate consequences before engaging in a behavior. Anticipating outcomes is often influenced by one's previous experiences. Expectancies are rooted in past experiences. However, unlike expectancies, they are more personalized as they depend on the significance an individual places on a specific outcome.

Self-efficacy is a concept that revolves around an individual's confidence in their ability to effectively carry out a particular behavior. Self-efficacy stands out from other theories as it was the first to introduce this concept. However, other theories, like the Theory of Planned Behavior by Ajzen, have since incorporated or introduced this construct at a later time. Self-efficacy is influenced by more than just a person's overall capabilities or qualities. It is also affected by individual characteristics and the surrounding environment, including barriers and facilitators.

3.4.1. Limitations Related to SCT

There are several limitations to consider when examining the model:

1. The idea suggests that when the environment undergoes constant change, it may not always result in a corresponding change in the individual.
2. The theory is not presented as a comprehensive system, but rather in a concise manner, highlighting the interplay between individuals, their behavior, and the environment (Bussey & Bandura, 1999). Nevertheless, there remains a level of uncertainty surrounding the significant impact that each of these factors has on actual behavior and how they interact with one another.
3. The theory primarily emphasizes learning processes, disregarding the significant influence of biological and hormonal predispositions on human behavior, which are not easily modified by experience and expectations.

3.5. Ecological Model

There are a variety of effective models that have been proven to encourage behavioral modifications, rather than just a single "ecological model". These models utilize principles from behavior modification and apply them to the field of biology. In the field of biological ecology, it is acknowledged that there are interactions between individuals within a species and other living things in communities, as well as between physical and abiotic variables within an ecosystem (Hovell, Wahlgren, & Gehrman, 2002). Emergent features are observed at all levels of organization within ecological systems due to the interactions between different components.

3.5.1. Characteristics of Ecological Models

It is important to consider that behaviors can be influenced by various factors. These factors can include personal experiences and attitudes, family and cultural traditions, workplace procedures, local community resources such as walking trails in parks, and even public policies like smoking laws.

It is important to consider the interactions that take place at different levels within a system. For example, the act of viewing a television advertisement promoting a government-funded smoking cessation program. This experience has the potential to influence a smoker's perspective on the habit of smoking.

Domain specificity is a crucial characteristic that cannot be overlooked. It is important to consider the various effects on an individual's smoking habits compared to their eating, exercise, or illness-prevention habits, especially in the field of public health. Understanding the fundamental principles of ecological models can greatly enhance our thought process, even when we are examining different specific aspects. This adaptability is what makes ecological models invaluable in the ever-evolving field of STEM education.

Effective interventions should aim to address multiple levels of the system. Asking faculty to adopt a new teaching method that is both recognized and incentivized by the university can be quite challenging. This is especially true when the university's policies and organizational structure continue to reward the traditional teaching approach.

3.5.2. Limitations and Assumptions

Ecological models are intentionally designed to be adaptable and specific to different situations. Therefore, it is important to conduct local research in order to pinpoint the specific factors that influence behavior, even though broader categories such as contextual, social, or personal aspects can provide some assistance in our analysis (Hovell, Wahlgren, & Gehrman, 2002). These models operate under the assumption that a change agent possesses the necessary authority to implement changes across all levels of the system. This authority is typically derived from public health domains, such as enacting a policy change at a high level to ban the use of tobacco. While implementing a multi-level strategy that is generally recommended, it is important to acknowledge that there are instances where external factors (e.g., influence of an accrediting body) can impact faculty conduct in ways that are beyond your control. It is important to note that modifying one's environment can potentially foster a shift in behavior, although it is not a foolproof method.

3.6. The Theory of Self-Determination

Self-determination refers to an individual's ability to autonomously make decisions and manage their own life. Being self-resolved means having a greater sense of control over your life, as opposed to feeling restricted by others' decisions. It conveys that individuals are motivated to grow and transform by three inherent (and universal) psychological needs. The concept of intrinsic motivation (engaging in activities for the inherent reward of the behavior itself) plays a significant role in this theory.

Deci and Ryan (2012) argue that self-determination plays a crucial role in psychology as it influences mental well-being and overall prosperity. Promoting self-determination is also a growing effective approach when working with specific populations, such as individuals with intellectual disabilities.

The self-determination hypothesis aims to understand how having a strong sense of self-resolve influences motivation. It suggests that individuals are more motivated to take action when they believe that their actions will have a meaningful impact on the outcome. The self-determination hypothesis suggests that individuals can achieve self-determination when their needs for competence, relatedness, and autonomy are fulfilled.

3.6.1. Principles Underlying Self-Determination

According to Deci and Ryan (2012), the self-determination hypothesis is based on two main assumptions:

1. Conduct is driven by the need for development. The central assumption of the self-determination hypothesis is that individuals are inherently motivated to achieve personal growth and progress. Developing resilience and embracing new experiences are essential for cultivating a lasting sense of self.
2. Autonomy in finding inspiration holds great importance. While external rewards such as money, prizes, and recognition often motivate individuals to take action (referred to as extrinsic motivation), self-determination theory primarily focuses on internal sources of motivation, such as a desire to acquire knowledge or autonomy (intrinsic motivation).

3.6.2. Components of Self-Determination

According to the self-determination hypothesis, individuals must experience the following in order to achieve their goals:

- **Autonomy:** Individuals require a sense of control over their own actions and goals. The ability to make an immediate decision that will result in substantial change has a profound effect in helping individuals who are not completely settled.

- **Competence:** Individuals must attain proficiency in tasks and master diverse skills. When individuals believe they possess the necessary skills for success, they are more likely to take actions that will help them achieve their goals.
- **Association or Relatedness:** Individuals require a sense of belonging and connection to others.

3.6.3. The Functioning of the Self-Determination Hypothesis

It is crucial to comprehend that the cognitive advancement portrayed by the self-determination hypothesis does not happen spontaneously. While individuals may have a predisposition towards such growth, it necessitates a continuous supply of nourishment. Assistance in social matters is crucial. By establishing and maintaining relationships and effectively exchanging information with others, we have the ability to either foster or hinder our own success and understanding of ourselves.

Variables that either facilitate or impede the essential components necessary for growth include:

- Occasionally, external influences can diminish one's self-motivation.
- Granting individuals external accolades for inherently motivated behavior can undermine autonomy.
- As external rewards increasingly limit people's behavior, they begin to feel less control over their actions and their intrinsic motivation decreases.

Constructive feedback can facilitate self-determination (Deci & Ryan, 2012). Providing candid and constructive feedback on an individual's performance can enhance intrinsic motivation. This type of criticism helps individuals develop a greater sense of readiness, which is an essential prerequisite for self-improvement.

3.6.4. Illustration of Self-Determination

Imagine an individual who fails to complete a crucial task at work. If this person possesses a high level of self-determination, they will acknowledge their weakness, recognize their ability to effectively rectify the problem, and take action to address the mistake. If the person in question lacked self-determination, they might instead seek out various things to blame. They could justify, assign blame elsewhere, or refuse to acknowledge their own responsibility in failing to complete the task on time. Primarily, it is likely that an individual lacking self-determination will not be motivated to rectify the mistake. Assuming all factors are equal, individuals may experience a sense of vulnerability in being unable to influence or have any significant impact on the current situation.

3.7. Social Ecological Model

The development of socio-biological models aim to enhance our understanding of the complex relationships between individuals and their environment. Socioecological models were introduced to urban studies by sociologists from The Chicago School in response to the limited scope of research conducted by developmental psychologists. These models bridge the gap between social theories that focus on small settings and anthropological theories.

Wold and Mittelmark (2018) identified the key components of the social ecological model as follows (Figure 3.5):

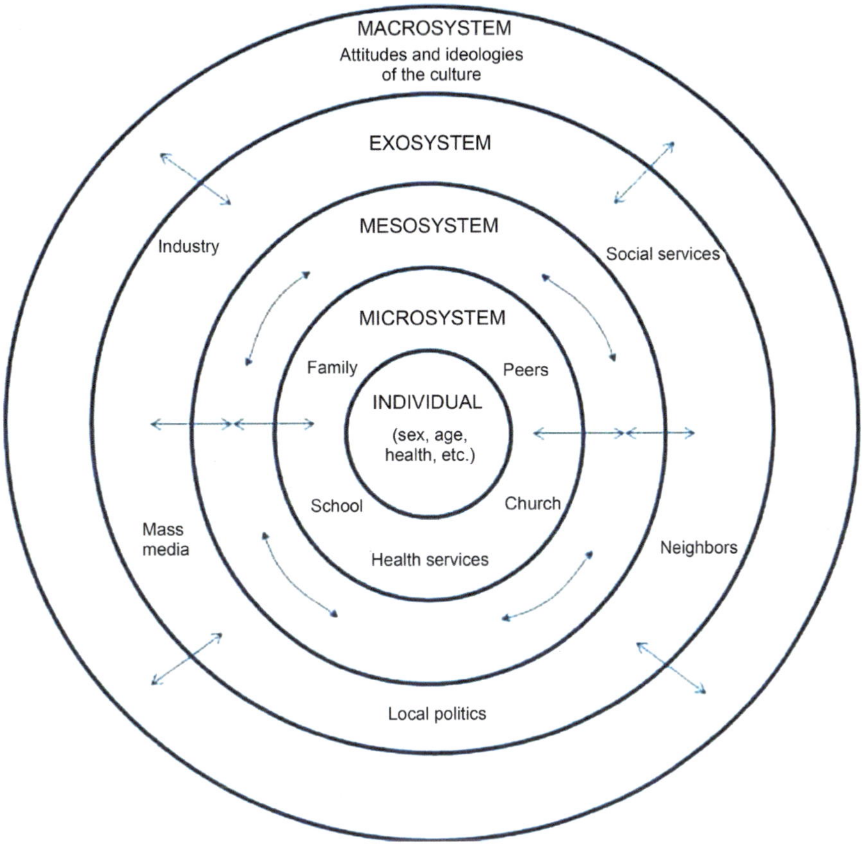

Figure 3.5. *Ecological framework for human development.*

Source: Social Ecological Model (2024).

3.7.1. Microsystem

The microsystem is the layer closest to the child and encompasses the patterns that the young individual directly interacts with. The microsystem encompasses the connections and interactions a child has with their immediate surroundings, such as their family, school, neighborhood, or childcare environments. At the microsystem level, the impacts that go both ways are particularly significant and have a strong influence on the child. Regardless, it is important to note that external communications can still have an impact on internal strategies. This center climate serves as the perfect environment for children to begin their journey of learning about the world. Being the child's most intimate learning environment, it provides them with a frame of reference for the world. The microsystem can serve as a crucial focal point for the child or potentially become a collection of distressing memories. The true significance of this foundational network of connections with family for the child lies in their ability to cultivate trust and a sense of belonging with their loved ones. The family serves as the child's primary microsystem for learning how to navigate life.

3.7.2. Mesosystem

Mesosystems involve the integration of multiple frameworks that encompass the lives of children, parents, and families. Mesosystems illustrate the connection between the structures of the child's microsystem. For example, the connection between the child's teacher and his/her parents, church, and community, all represent mesosystems.

3.7.3. Exosystem

The exosystem describes the larger social framework in which the child does not directly operate. The designs in this layer have a significant impact on the child's development as they interact with various elements in their microsystem. Parent work environment schedules and local area-based family resources serve as examples. Children may not be directly engaged at this level, but they do experience the positive or negative impact involved in their interactions with their own system. There are several key factors that can have a significant impact on young people through their family. These factors include:

- The school environment and the friends they interact with
- The workplace of their parents
- The social networks within their family
- The community they live in
- Local politics and industry

3.7.4. Macrosystem

The macrosystem refers to the larger social setting that encompasses various perspectives and social circumstances within the culture in which the child is situated. Macrosystems are often used to illustrate the social or cultural context of various cultural groups, such as social classes, ethnic groups, or religious affiliations. The furthest layer in the youngster's current circumstance is this layer. The impacts of larger standards set by the macrosystem have a cascading effect throughout the interactions of all other layers. The macrosystem has a significant influence on the way we conduct our relationships, including the what, how, when, and where.

For example, a program such as Women, Infants, and Children (WIC) can have a significant impact on a young mother by providing healthcare, nutrition, and other educational resources. It could enhance her life, allowing her to become more empowered and nurturing towards her newborn. In this model, the absence of a strong foundation of beliefs, policies, and support for families exposes children and their parents to significant harm and deterioration.

3.7.5. Chronosystem

The chronosystem encompasses the element of time as it interacts with a child's environment. Components within this framework can exist in different contexts. For instance, there are external components, such as the planning involved in a parent's passing. On the other hand, there are internal components, like the physiological changes that occur during a child's development. It is important to highlight the relational peculiarities within each system in a verifiable setting.

Here are a few models:

- Political and financial strategies that emphasize the importance of parents' jobs in their children's development, such as Early Advantage of Kids programs.
- Promoting cultural mindsets that value the work done for the benefit of young people at all levels: parents, teachers, extended family, mentors, employers, politicians.

In the field of public health promotion, it is crucial to identify key areas of impact and the factors that can facilitate the successful implementation of health-promoting interventions within organizations. This involves integrating both individual-focused and environment-based components into comprehensive health promotion programs, as well as assessing the long-term scope and sustainability of intervention outcomes. The premise of intercession projects is to address various issues such as harassment, obesity, overeating, and lack of physical activity. These interventions utilize the social ecological model as a framework, which includes extensive media campaigns, social marketing, and skills development.

3.8. Health Action Process Model

The Health Action Process Approach (HAPA) proposes that the adoption, initiation, and maintenance of health behaviors should be viewed as a sequential process, comprising of a motivation phase and a volition phase. There is another way to break down the latter, which involves three distinct phases - planning, action, and maintenance. Perceived self-efficacy is said to have a significant impact throughout various stages, alongside other cognitive factors (Zhang et al., 2019).

As an illustration, risk perceptions play a crucial role in initiating a thoughtful process during the early stages of motivation, but their influence does not go beyond that. In the realm of motivation, outcome expectancies play a significant role. They come into play when individuals weigh the potential benefits and drawbacks of certain behaviors. However, once a personal decision has been made, their ability to predict outcomes diminishes. However, without a strong belief in one's own capabilities, one will struggle to adopt, initiate, and maintain a desired action (Figure 3.6).

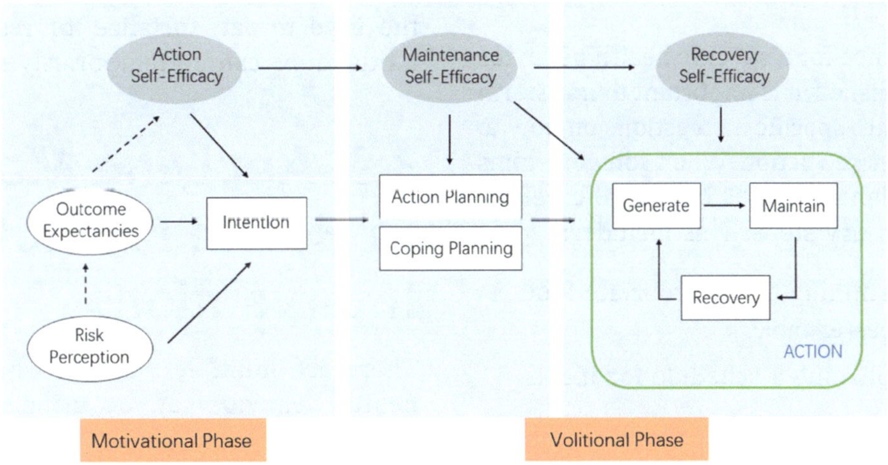

Figure 3.6. *Detailed path in the HAPA model.*

Source: Wu et al. (2022).

3.8.1. Motivation

During the motivation phase, individuals make a conscious decision to either adopt preventive measures or change risky behaviors in favor of more favorable ones. Self-efficacy and expectation of outcomes are considered to be the main factors that determine one's intentions. In the majority of previous models, the two predictors are considered unrelated. However, there could be a more practical and informal request among them. Anticipating results is crucial in determining one's self-confidence, as people often form assumptions about the potential outcomes of their actions before considering whether they can actually follow through. If self-efficacy is identified as a mediator between intention and outcome expectations, the impact of outcome expectancy on intention may be reduced. The research findings on this issue are highly conflicting, presenting both perspectives as viable options for driving change. In situations where individuals are not actively engaged in the activity they are contemplating, it is believed that outcome expectations may have a stronger influence than self-efficacy. Only when a sufficient level of engagement is reached does self-sufficiency gain more influence in determining a goal.

3.8.2. Volition

Once a preference for a specific health behavior has been established, it is important to transform the intention into specific instructions on how to perform the desired action. When someone aims to achieve weight loss, it is crucial to carefully plan the necessary steps. This includes:

- Determining the appropriate food choices to make
- Establishing a schedule for meals
- Deciding on the frequency of eating
- Selecting suitable workout times and locations
- Considering the possibility of quitting smoking as well

By considering a range of subordinate expectations and activity plans, a global objective can be established. These plans include proximal goals and calculations of action clusters. The volition interaction is minimally influenced by result anticipations but significantly impacted by self-viability. This is because the quantity and quality of activity plans are determined by one's perceived skill and experience. Self-adequacy convictions have a significant impact on the mental development of explicit activity plans. This is achieved by envisioning situations that could potentially lead to the fulfillment of objectives. Without these pre-action thoughts, individuals would make impulsive decisions without any guidance on how to allocate their available resources. Once an activity has been initiated, it is essential to adhere to certain perceptions in order to maintain momentum. It is crucial to ensure that conflicting intentions do not disrupt or prematurely halt the execution of a behavior. The meta-mental movement aims to complete the necessary task and suppress any distracting secondary inclinations. As an example, engaging in regular physical activity requires individuals to employ self-regulation techniques to sustain their effort and determination, while also resisting other competing motivations like the urge to eat, socialize, or rest, until these motivations can be temporarily set aside.

3.9. Applying Models to Health Promotion Interventions

There are multiple ways in which models of health behavior can be utilized to enhance individuals' overall well-being.

- **Health Belief Model:** According to research conducted by Bergeron et al. (2017), individuals are more inclined to take proactive measures in preventing or managing health conditions when they have a perception of the potential risks involved. Health promotion utilizes the Health Belief Model to customize messages that effectively target these factors. As an illustration:

- **Educational Campaigns:** One effective strategy is to conduct educational campaigns that emphasize the serious health risks associated with behaviors such as drinking and smoking. By raising awareness about the severity of related diseases, these campaigns can serve as a powerful motivator for individuals to quit those behaviors.
- **Screening Programs:** Highlighting the advantages of early detection for cancer prevention.

- **Theory of Planned Behavior:** The theory of planned behavior is commonly employed to modify health behaviors, alter social norms, and empower individuals to effectively change their behavior.
- **Social Cognitive Theory:** One effective approach is to utilize role models to demonstrate positive behaviors and establish stable environments that facilitate behavior change.
- **The Transtheoretical Model:** This is a widely used framework in psychology and behavior change. It provides a comprehensive understanding of how individuals progress through different stages when making a change in their behavior. This model has been extensively studied and has proven to be effective in various fields, such as addiction treatment and health promotion. By understanding the different stages of change, professionals can tailor interventions and support provided to individuals at each stage.

In practical terms, these models serve as a guide for promoting well-being interventions, ensuring that our efforts are based on evidence, while being targeted and effective. Through a comprehensive understanding of theories on behavior change, we can foster the development of more cohesive communities and empower individuals to make informed decisions.

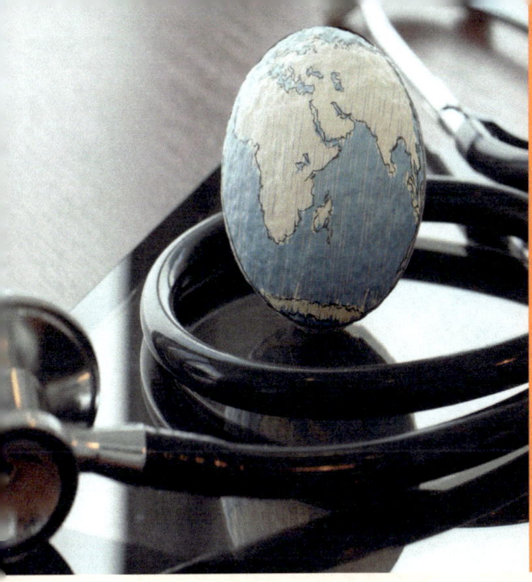

Chapter 4

HEALTH PROMOTION IN VARIOUS SETTINGS

Contents

4.1. Workplace Health Promotion

Workplace Health Promotion involves the utilization of health promotion resources by employers, employees, and society to improve the health and well-being of individuals. Along with the strategic components listed below, figure 4.1 outlines the steps to accomplish WHP.

- Implementing a strategy that involves cultivating a positive work environment and improving the overall structure and conditions of the workplace.

- Facilitating active engagement.
- Promoting individual growth.
- Implementation of an organizational philosophy aimed at improving the overall health status of the workforce.
- Systematically conveying important information to employees and the overall policies and practices related to health at workplace.
- Establishing a culture that fosters the concept of a collaborative work environment
- Implementing measures to minimize the amount of effort employees need to exert in order to make healthy choices.

Some examples of components and strategies for workplace health programs include:

- Health education classes.
- The close proximity to health and fitness gyms.
- Organizational policy regarding healthy behaviors, such as a policy that prohibits the use of tobacco in workplace.
- Health insurance coverage on the utilization of appropriate preventive screenings among employees.
- A conducive work environment: This entails establishing a work environment that promotes good health by providing access to nutritious food options, either through vending machines or the cafeteria. An optimal and secure working environment devoid of acknowledged risks, with a mechanism to identify and manage emerging risks.

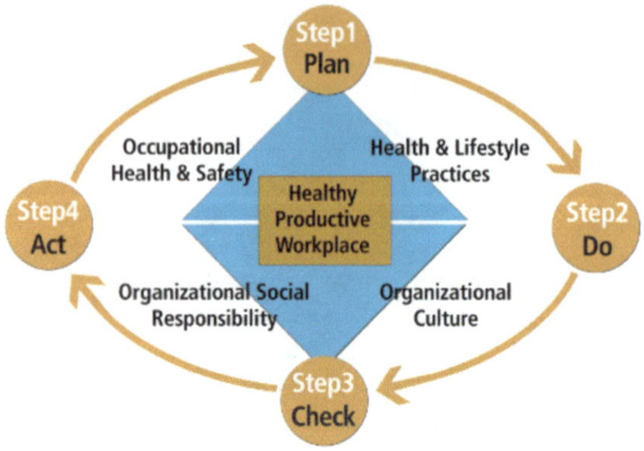

Figure 4.1. *The comprehensive workplace health (CWH) model.*

Source: Theme Grill (2021).

4.1.1. The Impact of Workplace Health Programs on Employee Health and Productivity

Workplace health programs can have a positive impact on individuals at both the individual or micro level and on the overall structure or macro level of an organization. The effectiveness of these programs can also vary depending on the type of organization and the specific characteristics of the employees.

At the individual level, workplace health programs can directly impact employees by influencing their health behaviors, the likelihood of developing a disease, and their current state of health (Gorgenyi-Hegyes, Nathan, & Fekete-Farkas, 2021).

Workplace health programs are pertinent to organizations and have the potential to impact various aspects, including healthcare expenses, work absenteeism, productivity improvement, employee recruitment and retention, organizational culture, and employee morale.

Gorgenyi-Hegyes, Nathan, and Fekete-Farkas (2021) outline four key steps in the systematic development of a workplace health promotion program:

Step 1: Conduct a Comprehensive Evaluation of the Health and Safety Conditions in the Workplace

An effective workplace health program should be tailored to the specific needs of employees at each worksite, taking into account the employee population and the goals of both individuals and the organization. The collection of this information can be initiated by initially implementing a workplace health assessment phase. An assessment should strive to comprehensively depict the various factors that impact employee health, such as socio-economic factors like occupational environments and personal lifestyles. Factors that shape the behavior of knowledge sharing within an organization include its organizational culture and practices. The role of knowledge attributes job context and social support in mediating the correlation between workplace practices, culture, and policies. Informal methods of gathering employee feedback include engaging in conversations with employees, soliciting input or opinions through methods such as placing a token in a box labeled 'opinion' or 'suggestion', or sending an email to request ideas. Formal methods involve having employees complete specific instruments such as an employee health survey, an environmental audit, or a questionnaire for workplace assessment.

Step 2: Program Design and Development

Any decisions regarding the implementation of programs, policies, benefits, or supports at the worksite must be preceded by a period of planning. The proposed program requires a basic infrastructure or governance system to organize and carry out health-promotion activities. This system can be developed during the planning stage. It is recognized that the size of the company, its sector, or its geographic location may affect the scale and complexity of each step. The governance structure of the business entity ensures that both strategic and operational inputs are provided to drive the program elements and bring them into existence. Organizational strategies provide the framework for achieving the fundamental objectives of the program, addressing employee well-being in a productive and efficient manner, and managing business resources with ethical considerations.

Step 3: Executing the Program

Employers often prioritize individualistic behaviors when seeking to improve the health of their workers. For instance, reducing the intake of saturated fat, maintaining a healthy weight, and refraining from smoking are additional behaviors that each contribute to improved health. However, it is essential to comprehend that good health encompasses more than just physical fitness. It also encompasses the environments in which individuals work, play, and socialize. Both employees and employers possess significant influence over the workplace, enabling them to shape conditions that foster good health and prevent diseases. Modifying the environment has a simultaneous impact on the workforce and facilitates the adoption of beneficial behaviors (either when such behaviors are deemed acceptable or with the backing of workplace regulations). Therefore, it is imperative that the comprehensive workplace health program integrates a combination of individual and organizational level strategies and interventions to improve health.

Step 4: Assess the Effect by Conducting an Evaluation

Ultimately, the workplace should evaluate the efficacy of the implemented programs, policies, benefits, or environmental supports. It is imperative to assess the long-term viability of the workplace health program, including its ability to sustain effectiveness over time, employee and management perceptions, and return on investment. Assessments are regarded as a fundamental aspect of public health, and program evaluation is widely acknowledged as a cornerstone of effective evaluation methodology. However, adhering to proper evaluation protocols typically entails investing both time and money – resulting in the generation of findings that are ultimately not utilized for program enhancement. The evaluation should focus on several key aspects:

- Firstly, the choice of questions should be pertinent and meaningful to both the users of the evaluation and the decision-making processes that rely on it.
- Secondly, the evaluation should be applied in a way that allows for re-entry into the quality improvement cycle. This means that any weaknesses identified should be used to strengthen or improve existing activities.
- Additionally, any gaps or shortcomings should be identified for further investigation.
- Lastly, the evaluation should assess the efficiency and effectiveness of the resources invested.

4.2. Health Promotion Activities Implemented Within Schools

A health promoting school is a school that is dedicated to consistently supporting the physical environment of the school as a space for living, learning, and working. An institution that actively promotes and prioritizes the well-being and health of its students and staff ensures the following:

1. Enhances well-being and facilitates the acquisition of knowledge through all available methods in the present era.
2. Engages in the activities of convincing health and education authorities, teachers' unions, teachers, students, parents, healthcare providers, and other community leaders to prioritize the promotion of a healthy environment within the school.
3. Promotes a conducive and beneficial environment within schools, providing comprehensive health education, establishing and enhancing school health services and initiatives that promote collaboration between schools and communities. Additionally, it aims to implement programs that promote the well-being of school staff, ensuring proper nutrition and food hygiene, providing opportunities for physical education and recreational activities, and offering counseling, social support, and mental health promotion initiatives.
4. Implements and ensures equitable practices that prioritize the well-being and dignity of individuals. Provides multiple chances for individuals to succeed and values their efforts and commendable attempts as much as actual achievements.
5. Aims to enhance the well-being of school staff, students' family members, and neighbors by actively sharing health and education-related information with community leaders.

Small children are crucial members of primary communities, as over 90% of all children aged 5–15 years are enrolled in primary schools worldwide (Bramantoro et al., 2021). School-based interventions target a wide range of children and parents who belong to various diverse categories. Teachers and school nurses are the most suitable individuals to take action in promoting health, preventing illnesses, and intervening early in health issues that may impede a child's academic achievement. Schools have been found to provide optimal conditions for implementing regulations that reduce the risks of noncommunicable diseases and promote overall health while preventing unhealthy behaviors. Ultimately, the research findings indicate that it is crucial to cultivate social-emotional strengths and enhance social-emotional skills. Issues such as self-knowledge, self-esteem, emotional self-regulation, and positive assertiveness skills serve as protective factors against behavioral difficulties, including illegal and deviant behaviors, violent and aggressive behaviors, substance abuse, bullying, problematic internet use, and school dropouts among primary school children and adolescents (Bramantoro et al., 2021). Notably, research has shown that psycho-educational interventions aimed at promoting well-being in schools have been associated with improved behavior outcomes, socio-emotional competence, higher academic achievement and graduation rates, and a positive overall school climate.

4.3. Promotion of Community Health

Health promotion in community health involves organizing activities that empower individuals and groups in communities to take action and have control over their health. The term "health promotion" encompasses initiatives and endeavors aimed at fostering optimal health, mitigating health hazards, injuries, and associated factors, and enhancing the overall well-being of the community (Cislaghi et al., 2019). Health promotion focuses on employing strategies to influence social, economic, environmental, and behavioral factors in order to enhance overall health conditions.

4.3.1. Essential Elements of Health Promotion in Community

Education and awareness: The process of health promotion usually begins by providing information and raising awareness among the general population about the risks associated with health, promoting healthy behaviors, and highlighting the benefits of adopting a healthy lifestyle. This may entail engaging in dialog with audiences in community workshops or health campaigns and disseminating information through pamphlets and similar means.

- **Behavior Modification:** Health promotion educates individuals on how to take initiative and make behavioral enhancements in their lives. For instance, promoting cessation and discouraging the consumption of cigarettes and other tobacco products, reducing alcohol consumption, engaging in regular physical exercise, adopting a healthy diet, and practicing safe sexual behavior, among other things.
- **Preventive Services:** Preventive services are an integral part of health promotion and encompass access to vaccinations, cancer screenings (which can be accessed within a few weeks or months), and regular check-ups. These groups are actively mobilized to enhance the accessibility and utilization of these services.
- **Community Engagement:** The notion that 'health is personal' is crucial in health promotion as it necessitates active involvement from community members. It also entails the ability of communities to identify and address specific challenges they encounter in their daily lives and determine

effective solutions for them. Additionally, there are various forms of participation, such as health committees, support groups, and advocacy activities.

- **Policy and Environmental Changes:** This is integral to health promotion, as it goes beyond simply encouraging individuals to change their behaviors. Instead, it emphasizes the importance of addressing the wider social and physical environment that impacts health. This could involve advocating for the adoption of smoking regulations or promoting policies that support healthy lifestyles, such as efficient transportation systems.
- **Social Determinants of Health:** Recognizing the significance of social factors such as income, education, housing, and health in health promotion is crucial. Activities may encompass efforts aimed at mitigating poverty and/or advocating for social equity.
- **Empowerment and Capacity Building:** Health promotion involves strengthening the capabilities of individuals and communities to enhance their own health. This entails the establishment of consciousness, acquiring novel knowledge such as in the realm of health, and the facilitation of resources for the process of making informed choices.

4.3.2. Methods for Enhancing the Well-Being of the Local Population

- **Community Needs Assessment:** As a component of your community health education plan, conduct a thorough and extensive evaluation of the needs of the community (community health needs assessment). This could involve employing surveys, focus groups, or data assimilation techniques to ascertain the most pressing health issues.
- **Collaboration and Partnerships:** Establish strategic partnerships with other entities within the public health system, such as healthcare facilities, patient-centered centers, educational institutions, workplaces, and religious institutions (Cislaghi et al., 2019). Collaboration among practitioners is crucial for coordinating health programs and improving the overall effectiveness of comprehensive health initiatives within a society.
- **Health Promotion and Education:** Implement an educational strategy aimed at enhancing the community's awareness and adoption of healthier lifestyle choices, preventing diseases, and increasing their knowledge of available healthcare resources. These can manifest as seminars, informational booths, educational and awareness campaigns on social media, or public health announcements.
- **Healthy Environments:** Strives to create conducive surroundings that promote good health, offering opportunities for physical exercise through the use of parks and recreational facilities, access to affordable and nutritious foods, and the provision of cycling paths and

safe walking routes. This promotes the adoption of exercise and the inclusion of nutritious foods.

4.4. The Role of Healthcare Settings in Promoting Health

The implementation of health promotion strategies in healthcare settings holds significant potential and is driven by the field of public health. Clinics account for approximately 40% to 70% of public medical care utilization and typically employ around 1% to 3% of the workforce (D'Andreamatteo et al., 2015). These operational locations are characterized by specific physical, synthetic, organic, and psychosocial factors that pose risks. Surprisingly, in medical clinics (organizations that aim to restore health), the identification of factors that endanger the well-being of their staff is poorly developed. Emergency clinics can also have a lasting impact on the behavior of patients and family members, who are more open to health advice when they are experiencing illness.

With the increasing prevalence of chronic diseases worldwide and low adherence to treatment, therapeutic education is becoming a significant concern. The majority of emergency clinic therapies aim to enhance the quality of life for patients rather than providing a cure. In order to uphold this standard, it is imperative that patients and their loved ones are adequately equipped and informed for their release. Hospitals produce a substantial amount of waste and dangerous substances. Implementing health promotion strategies can effectively mitigate environmental pollution in hospitals. Collaborating with other institutions and professionals can optimize care coordination. Hospitals serve as research and teaching institutions, generating and sharing a significant amount of knowledge. This knowledge can influence local health systems and professional practices in other areas. Despite the initial belief that hospitals could do more for people's health, there is now substantial evidence supporting the effectiveness of health promotion activities in hospitals. Furthermore, the implementation of health promotion activities within quality improvement programs will have a greater impact on the well-being of individuals and communities. Health promotion in hospitals encompasses interventions targeting both individuals (patients and staff) as well as structures and processes. The use of quantitative methodology is crucial in evaluating various interventions. It is not feasible to conduct a prospective controlled trial to demonstrate the effects of a comprehensive hospital program for health promotion, a quality management plan, or an accreditation program. However, specific interventions such as inducing tobacco cessation or alcohol abstinence before planned surgery have been unquestionably documented in randomized controlled trials (D'Andreamatteo et al., 2015). The quantitative approach also quantifies the value of more intricate interventions such as rehabilitation programs. The evaluation of cycles and designs in a program should be conducted using a subjective methodology, allowing for the interpretation of results and the inclusion of emotional or political judgments.

Despite limited legislative support in many member countries, the International Network of Health Promoting Hospitals has experienced a consistent growth in the number of hospitals and countries joining. The organization was expanded based on philosophical principles and values, but continues to lack rules or substantial projects for implementing exercises in certain clinics. Additionally, there is still a lack of information regarding the extent and nature of health promotion activities being carried out in these clinics. Furthermore, there is a dearth of information concerning the rationales behind hospitals' decision to join the network (D'Andreamatteo et al., 2015). Wellbeing promotion must demonstrate its worthiness of the investment. Currently, we have limited evidence to suggest that an HPH (High Pressure Homogenization) is superior to a non-HPH method. Only limited resources have been allocated to enhance health promotion. Therefore, there is no valid reason to believe that it had a negative impact on hospital operations by diverting resources from the core functions of the hospital.

4.5. Promotion of Global Health

As globalization increasingly impacts various aspects of our lives, we are beginning to understand how factors that extend beyond the national boundaries of individual countries are affecting the factors that determine health and well-being outcomes.

The influence on health determinants, status, and outcomes cannot be exclusively accomplished through actions taken at the national level, given the fact that numerous health risks and opportunities are progressively becoming globalized (Dodgson, Lee, & Drager, 2017). The surge in cross-border flows of people, ideas, labor, and goods necessitates a reevaluation of the principles and frameworks that govern health policy and practice (Figure 4.2).

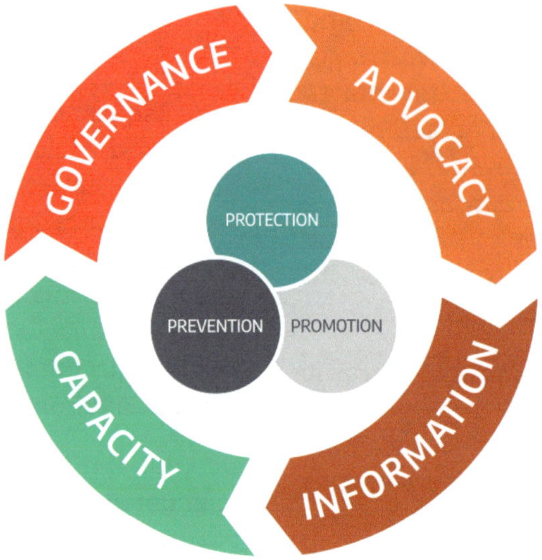

Figure 4.2. *The global charter for the public's health.*

Source: The Global Charter for the Public's Health | WFPHA, (n.d).

Given the extent to which globalization necessitates global management technology for health, it is necessary to reassess conventional approaches to health promotion. It is necessary to understand how globalization (the increasing flow of people, money, information, and ideas across borders) is impacting the process of empowering individuals to gain control over and improve their well-being.

For instance, to enhance sexual health, it may be imperative to focus more on the changing trends of migration, tourism, displaced populations, migrant workers, and other types of population movement within and among countries. The promotion of global brands by multinational corporations may need to be countered in order to promote the development of effective dietary plans. To advance tobacco control, it is necessary to implement measures to address the availability of illicit cigarettes and the targeting of emerging markets in low- and middle-income countries by multinational tobacco companies (Dodgson, Lee, & Drager, 2017).

The improvement of optimal living conditions may necessitate increased attention to the impact of large-scale agricultural production on urbanization and land availability.

Global health promotion can be defined as the systematic effort to empower individuals to have greater agency over their health and improve it within the context of a rapidly expanding world. Dodgson, Lee, and Drager (2017) argue that the challenge lies in establishing effective systems of governance to facilitate these initiatives. Wellbeing promotion, by definition, encompasses a wide range of social institutions, including governmental bodies and individual families. In practical terms, previous attempts to address global health issues have reflected the imbalanced nature of current institutions and deficiencies in their collaboration. When examining these models, we focus on the organizations and systems involved, the feasibility of these initiatives (strengths and weaknesses), and the lessons learned for future action.

4.6. Promotion of Health Using Digital Technology

The pervasive influence of technology is evident in various domains of our lives, ranging from the integration of health applications in smartphones to the utilization of activity trackers for monitoring heart rates. With the transition from the modern era to the data age, the field of wellbeing advancement is also progressing into a new technological era known as Digital Health Promotion (DHP) (Figure 4.3).

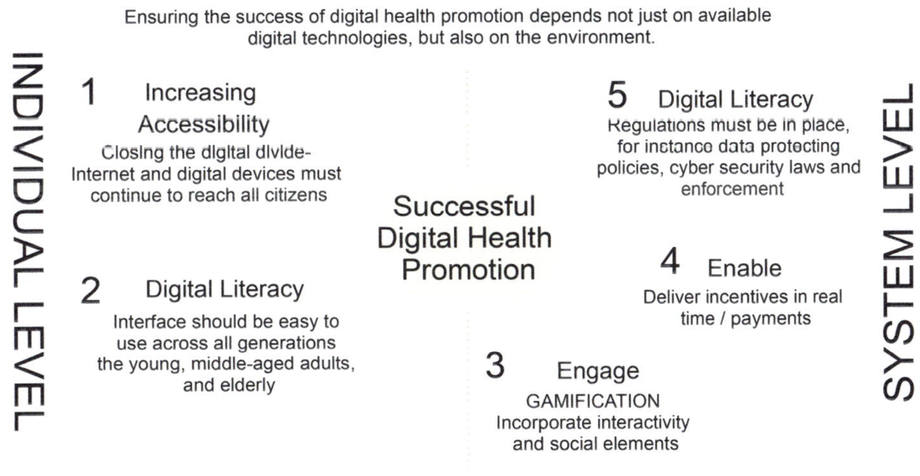

Figure 4.3. *Ecological system view of enabling digital health promotion.*

Source: Koh et al. (2021).

The Global Systems for Mobile Communications Association (GSMA), which represents mobile operators, estimated that in July 2020, there were 8.8 billion mobile connections and 5.1 billion unique smartphone subscribers. This represents a year-on-year growth of 6.2% and 3.72%, respectively (Mathews et al., 2019). These devices are a powerful tool for rapidly expanding efficient, personalized, and easily accessible health communication. The advent of computerized innovation has introduced new tools that are advancing population health by addressing numerous challenges related to access and cost. These technologies not only facilitate and reduce costs for health promoters to reach populations that are difficult to access (often in non-clinical settings such as homes or communities) but they also enable the customization of different types of health communication for specific subpopulations and even individuals.

Digitization not only provides cost-effective ways to reach people and create social change, but it also allows policy planners to have a detailed understanding of potential health promotion measures and their impact on the population as a whole by aggregating individual experiences at the population level (Mathews et al., 2019). These population-level findings can be utilized to enhance existing measures, identify underserved groups, and strategize the implementation of additional services such as in-person interventions.

4.6.1. Advantages of Digital Health Promotion

DHP enables the identification and assistance of individuals who are vulnerable and face challenges in seeking medical help due to social stigma or financial constraints. It also has the capability to reach communities that are remote or hard to access. Online platforms provide a discreet and anonymous way for individuals who are hesitant to engage in traditional therapy or counseling to seek support. Amidst the global Coronavirus pandemic and subsequent lockdowns in various regions, the rise of mental health issues has prompted many individuals to seek assistance through online platforms. In India, the number of online mental health applications, such as Your DOST, Wysa, and Mfine, has increased by 30% in terms of web-based solutions and call-ins. This increase can be attributed to the significant contribution of anxiety caused by the Coronavirus pandemic (Mathews et al., 2019). Similarly, individuals diagnosed with highly stigmatized diseases such as HIV/AIDS have also sought social support from various online platforms.

4.6.2. Difficulties and Danger

Despite the enthusiasm surrounding the benefits that DHP can offer, it remains a double-edged proposition. When implemented effectively, it can provide significant improvements in the field of health promotion, as demonstrated by the aforementioned standards. Nevertheless, it presents novel challenges that governments and public health organizations will have to tackle. These challenges encompass:

- **Challenges Regarding Privacy and the Subsequent Use of Data:** The highly sensitive nature of clinical information and its potential for optional utilization (and misuse) give rise to numerous concerns regarding data security, particularly for populations lacking specific privacy safeguards in place. Currently, the management of health information appears uncertain, as only about half of the countries recognized by the World Health Organization have regulations in place to protect personal health data (Mathews et al., 2019). In 2019, the Organization for Economic Co-operation and Development (OECD) published a health data governance framework that aims to safeguard privacy, personal health data, and data security, while also promoting the accessibility and utilization of personal health data for the benefit of public health.

- **Risks Related to Cybersecurity:** While online protection risks are not uncommon across various industries, the healthcare sector is particularly vulnerable due to the high value of health information. Although Facebook's suicide prevention program effectively detects and intervenes in potential cases, it also unavoidably identifies individuals at risk whose personal information may be vulnerable in the event of a cybersecurity breach. In September 2018, a significant data breach resulted in the compromise of over 50 million users' personal profiles. According to Mathews, et al., (2019), Facebook has not disclosed whether the compromised users in its suicide prevention algorithm were informed. This has raised concerns about Facebook's use of user data without consent, leading privacy experts to question whether Facebook can be considered a trustworthy platform, particularly when it comes to handling sensitive health information. Although Facebook collects and retains new health data related to mental health problems with the aim of preventing suicides, it is important to note that social media platforms, in general, are not obligated to comply with the same privacy regulations as healthcare providers.
- **Dissemination of Inaccurate Information and Intentionally Deceptive Statements:** General wellbeing data can often be intricate and nuanced, as professionals are hesitant to distort. However, this can confuse the general public or, even worse, be mistakenly perceived as a form of deception.

4.7. Health Promotion Policy and Advocacy

Advocacy for public health is commonly defined as the process of assuming political accountability for a particular goal or program, and acknowledged by some as a fundamental strategy for the well-being of the general population. The individuals you aim to communicate with are usually decision-makers, strategists, and program administrators who possess the ability to influence actions that can have a significant impact on a large number of people concurrently. Public health advocacy strategies promote the use of upstream methodology, recognizing that individual issues are often influenced by social circumstances. This approach involves addressing specific medical issues within the broader framework of social determinants that exist outside of individuals (Farrer et al., 2015). It also acknowledges the cultural diversity of public health problems and the challenges related to resources and logistics that are inherent in addressing these difficulties at the individual level. Although health promotion efforts such as smoking prevention, community-level interventions, and provider education are important for public health, some may view them as attempting to fix a problem with limited impact compared to the larger-scale interventions. Advocating for public health acknowledges the inherent political disparities within the field and emphasizes the importance of addressing social determinants of health as a crucial element in efforts to enhance the well-being of populations. In other words, advocating for general wellbeing is a crucial aspect of promoting optimal health conditions. If the goal of public health is to reduce the impact of health issues on society, effective treatment options could potentially alter the cultural forces that contribute to these problems. By disregarding the political and social dimensions of wellbeing, the practice of promoting general wellbeing is limited to merely avoiding risks and promoting individual factors.

The Ontario Health Promotion Resource System categorizes exercises into three levels: low, medium, and high intensity. Low-profile events may involve peaceful discussions, meetings with public officials, sharing of information, and the development of confidential briefings. Activities of a medium level involve continuous negotiations, drafting public briefs, engaging with opposition, acting as committee deputies, participating in meetings with selected authorities, and establishing strategic alliances with other groups (Farrer et al., 2015). In addition, writing letters to select authorities or newspapers. High intensity activities encompass public scrutiny, promotional activities, advertising campaigns, information dissemination, correspondence, and participation in demonstrations and rallies. Within this classification framework, various activities (such as interviewing officials and exchanging information) can be categorized into any of these classes.

Engaging in strategy promotion necessitates a distinct set of skills. The three essential competencies required for successful public health promotion are: 1) the ability to collaborate with various stakeholders, 2) strategic utilization of media, and 3) proficiency in conducting strategic analysis. It is necessary to concentrate on three main areas in order to develop this final skill (Farrer et al., 2015). The questions are: What is the issue? What is the nature or identity of the subject in question? Upon whom should the focus of change be directed? While often underestimated, the capacity to devise effective policy solutions is equally crucial as the ability to recognize the problems at hand in the context of advocating for the welfare of others. The capacity to accurately articulate problems as they are recognized is a crucial aspect of providing comprehensive support for overall well-being.

4.8. Religiously-Oriented Efforts to Promote Health and Well-Being

Religious leaders and faith communities are the largest and most well-organized universal institutions, representing the commitment of billions of followers and transcending barriers of race, class, and identity (Francis, 2016). Religious leaders possess a greater level of expertise in establishing and collaborating with global organizations compared to other members of the general population. Their expertise can greatly contribute to the global health promotion initiative. Religious leaders often hold the highest level of respect within their communities. Due to the trust bestowed upon them by their followers, Buddhist monks, nuns, imams, pastors, priests, punjaris, and leaders of other religious communities have a substantial influence on shaping attitudes, opinions, and behaviors. Religious leaders possess the authority to enhance consciousness and shape beliefs, actions, and customs, especially within the context of families and communities. They have the ability to shape societal values in alignment with religious doctrines. Religious leaders possess the capability (at these levels) to:

- Develop an understanding of the most effective methods for breastfeeding and encourage their religious communities to support and advocate for the rights of mothers to breastfeed.
- Inspire and instruct followers to embrace additional health-promoting practices that align with religious doctrines.
- Exhibit suitable and encouraging actions. For instance, female leaders who have infants or young children have the ability to nurse their babies, while male leaders and individuals known as "mothers of the church" can provide assistance and encouragement to their wives and daughters in breastfeeding.
- Enhance communication within families to establish a nurturing environment for the woman engaged in breastfeeding.
- Emphasize the husband's obligation to financially support his wife both during and after childbirth to families.
- Persuade communities and families to actively promote exclusive breastfeeding for the initial six months and to sustain breastfeeding for the first two years of a child's life.
- Create and organize breastfeeding support groups.
- Allocate dedicated areas within their premises to accommodate women who wish to breastfeed in seclusion during services and events, in accordance with prevailing norms or the preferences of the mothers.
- Disseminate information regarding the advantages of breastfeeding and the potential dangers of inadequate feeding methods to parents.
- Establish connections with religious leaders and other individuals in order to form a movement that promotes and advocates for the adoption of optimal breastfeeding practices.

Religious leaders can also promote and endorse public policies that protect the well-being of families, mothers, and children. Religious leaders can employ advocacy to:

- Enhance the voices of the disadvantaged when formulating regulations and strategies.
- Collaborate with the Ministry of Labor to facilitate exclusive breastfeeding for working women for a duration of six months.
- Influence the Ministry of Health to establish strategies for keeping the mother and child together in the immediate hours after birth to facilitate immediate initiation of breastfeeding.
- Support the crucial services of not providing recipes to mothers of infants under six months old who do not actually need them.
- Implement stricter regulations to impede businesses from marketing and selling baby formula to women who do not have a genuine need for it.

Religious leaders and faith communities are indeed capable of and actively pay attention to the rights of children (Francis, 2016). They are well-equipped to contribute their ethical and profound efforts to the local and global efforts to save lives by enhancing breastfeeding practices. Religious organizations can promote and communicate disease prevention and management programs in all communities. Examples of religious associations include temples, assembly halls, mosques, meeting houses, and various places of worship. They can be organized as assemblies, governmental institutions, or as independent entities.

Leaders of religious associations play a crucial role in the lives of individuals belonging to faith communities. The confidence in information sharing among faith-based organizations can be potent. Medical care experts recognize the crucial role of faith and spirituality in the perception of health, illness, and recovery.

Partnerships greatly enhance the effectiveness of faith-based interventions for disease prevention and management. Religious organizations can collaborate with established local assemblies to connect individuals with information, resources, and assistance. Religious individuals engaged in programming may include local community collaboration, screening, and diabetes education initiatives. Providing culturally competent care for different populations requires being sensitive to spirituality as a fundamental aspect of cultural identity.

4.9. Promotion of Health with a Focus on the Family

The family plays a crucial role in supporting and nurturing its members throughout different stages of life. Moreover, the family is an unmatched contributor to public health by promoting well-being and preventing illnesses. The family's ability to provide support, guidance, protection, education, and influence throughout one's life makes it a valuable starting point in promoting and maintaining both individual and collective health. It is also a crucial element in public health practice. Most individuals are part of families where each member is interconnected and influenced by one another, as explained by the family systems theory. However, recent changes in demographics, such as a larger proportion of older adults, an increasing number of multigenerational families, and more people living alone, require a significant shift in public health focus from the traditional emphasis on mothers and children to considering the broader family context. According to this theory, families are cohesive entities that operate as a system with distinct regulations and obligations (Kokorelias et al., 2019). Each family member exerts a substantial influence on the decisions made by other family members, and these decisions can result in enduring consequences that manifest as social inequalities, intergenerational destitution, and even the persistent physical and emotional ramifications of adverse childhood experiences.

Examples of health outcomes that would benefit from a family-based approach include:

- Genetic disorder testing for infants and children
- Rates of suicide and substance abuse among teenagers and young adults
- Noncommunicable diseases such as Alzheimer's and dementia among adult men

The increasing diversity of family configurations and social determinants of health underscores the complexity and importance of incorporating various family structures into public health. This offers significant potential for leveraging the family as a resource in promoting public health, while also recognizing the varying levels of protective factors and risks associated with different family configurations.

It is conceivable that families may lack awareness of the public health system and its potential to aid them in attaining their health and well-being goals. Mindful families may also have reservations about public health services due to limited knowledge or other factors. Obtaining the assurance of a parent or any member of a family involves:

- Refraining from disparaging opinions about the family's competence
- Resisting a conditional approach to collaboration
- Rejecting a condescending attitude of knowing better
- Acknowledging the rights and privacy of families and their need for autonomy in fulfilling their responsibilities

Public health practitioners must exhibit their regard and appreciation for the abilities, potential for development, and decision-making regarding health of every family. Ultimately, the remarkable alterations in family makeup, organization, schedules, and employment necessitate adaptability in order to address the potential health difficulties that families may encounter (Kokorelias et al., 2019). Exhibiting reverence and hopefulness can also manifest as cooperative family health policies or endorsing public health practices through a constructive, resourceful, and pertinent approach. This approach is significant in the context because numerous families place a high level of importance on their autonomy and confidentiality.

Children and young adults are likely to incorporate their own family experiences or traditions into their imagined relationships and future family decisions. Throughout their development, children and adolescents encounter various types of families and draw conclusions based on their observations, which may influence their expectations for their own future family. It is not always advisable to use one's own family experience as a model. Instead, providing assistance to children, teenagers, and young adults in acquiring positive behaviors from their immediate families or other individuals in close proximity is likely to be highly valued, particularly if the support addresses one or more universally desired needs. Directing attention towards positive family practices could serve as a favorable initial step. The composition of communities and populations, consisting of individuals and families, has a significant impact on the overall welfare of the local area. Family units are indispensable components of community systems and exert a substantial influence on health results. Various health behaviors, whether positive or negative, are inherently cultivated, upheld, and modified within the familial or domestic environment. Preliminary research indicates that family-oriented health promotion and disease prevention strategies are promising due to the fact that the family unit is considered both a resource and a priority group that necessitates preventative and curative services throughout all stages of life (Kokorelias et al., 2019). Health promotion practice often fails to fully utilize family health systems, despite the increasing number of successful initiatives. The lack of implementation in practice and policy has hindered the accumulation of substantial evidence for family health.

4.10. Culturally Customized Health Promotion

The acknowledgement that there is no universally applicable method for promoting well-being and preventing illness has led to the recognition of the importance of cultural factors in the creation of effective health interventions. Gaining a comprehensive understanding of social aspects and showing respect towards them is crucial for making interventions that resonate with individuals from diverse backgrounds. Cultural tailoring in the context of health interventions involves modifying programs to align with the specific cultural values, beliefs, and practices of a target population (Dickerson et al., 2020). Health behaviors are deeply ingrained in social environments and interventions should be tailored to resonate with diverse communities. Essentially, social fitting extends beyond surface-level differences, aiming to integrate cultural insights into the fundamental design of interventions. This ensures that health messages, strategies, and programs are not only linguistically appropriate but also culturally meaningful and scientifically relevant.

4.10.1. Health and Cultural Diversity

Human societies exhibit a wide range of cultural diversity, encompassing different ethnicities, languages, customs, and religions. This diversity is evident in works related to well-being, shaping individuals' perception of prosperity, illness, and healthcare. When it comes to the field of mental health, it is crucial to comprehend the intricate tapestry of social diversity in order to develop interventions that resonate with the unique backgrounds and experiences of diverse populations. The dynamics of segment movements, globalization, and relocation contribute to an increasingly diverse medical services landscape, necessitating a thorough understanding of cultural nuances in health promotion and disease prevention. Culture serves as a prominent lens through which individuals interpret health information, make decisions about healthcare utilization, and engage in health-promoting or risky behaviors. Social beliefs influence attitudes towards illness, perception of well-being and the causes of disease, and expectations of healthcare providers. Furthermore, cultural norms and the acceptability of specific health practices have an impact on communication styles in healthcare settings. It is crucial to recognize these effects in order to implement appropriate health interventions that align with societal values and are sensitive to how individuals from diverse cultural backgrounds navigate their health journey. Cultural differences have a significant impact on the health outcomes of diverse populations, and these differences are evident in various ways (Dickerson et al., 2020). For instance, dietary preferences influenced by cultural traditions may contribute to differences in nutrition-related health issues. Attitudes towards mental health, which can be influenced by cultural acceptance or stigma, can shape help-seeking behaviors. Differences in social communication styles can impact the interactions between patients and specialists, their compliance with medical advice, and ultimately, the effectiveness of treatment. To comprehend these components, one must consider the identification of specific areas where social adaptation can significantly impact health disparities, address the root causes of health inequalities, and promote equitable health outcomes among diverse communities.

Several models demonstrate the effectiveness of social integration in health interventions. Culturally tailored smoking cessation programs have shown enhanced efficacy among diverse populations by specifically targeting culturally specific triggers and incorporating culturally relevant messages. Customizing diabetes management interventions to the dietary preferences and cultural norms of specific ethnic groups has proven to be effective. Mindfulness practices, which are based on specific cultures, along with other mental health interventions that integrate cultural values and traditions, have shown greater acceptance and effectiveness (Dickerson et al., 2020). The importance of customizing interventions to align with the cultural contexts of diverse communities is demonstrated by these examples, leading to enhanced engagement and outcomes.

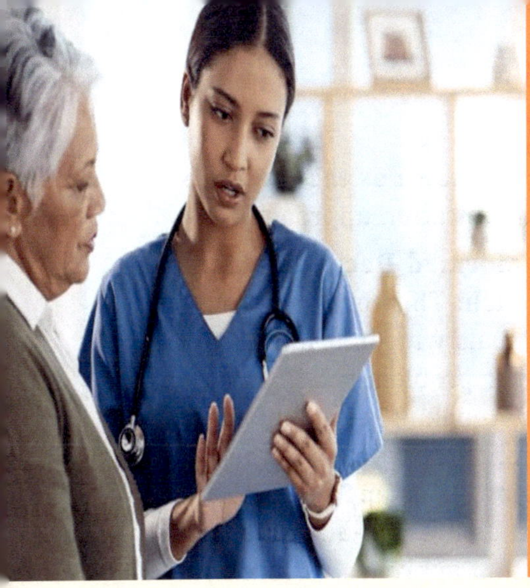

Chapter 5

HEALTH PROMOTION STRATEGIES

Contents

With health promotion, there are three fundamental strategies:

1. Advocacy for health
2. Facilitating universal access for all individuals: It involves the process of minimizing the occurrence of disease, preventing the onset of illness, and assisting individuals in overcoming health-related challenges. Gain greater autonomy and improve their well-being.
3. The mediator's role of navigating and resolving conflicts between multiple societal interests.

These three strategies can be implemented through various methods such as health education, behavior modification interventions, social marketing, media campaigns, policy formulation, environmental modification, community mobilization, and health coaching.

5.1. Health Education

Efforts to educate individuals about health-related matters are tailored based on the specific demographic being targeted. Health education provides information to individuals about specific health issues, including the potential benefits or drawbacks they may face. It also empowers them and promotes changes in their attitudes and behaviors in an appropriate context and at the right time (Koelen & Ban, 2023) (Figure 5.1).

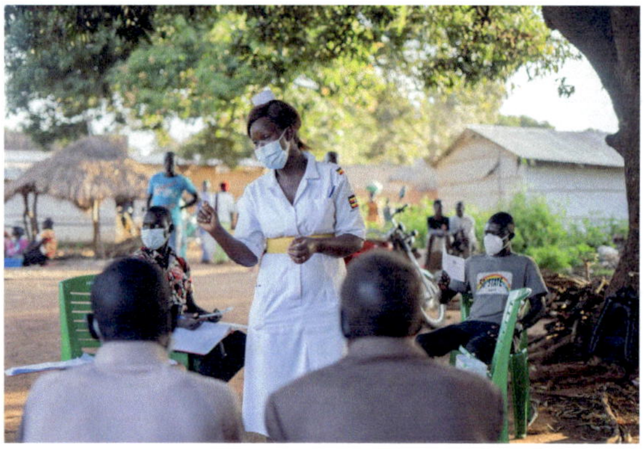

Figure 5.1. *Health education and public awareness for universal healthcare.*

Source: Borst (2021).

5.1.1. Health Education Approaches

Health education approaches can be categorized into different methods.

- **The Persuasion Approach:** This involves directly attempting to change the behaviors of others by guiding them towards the desired actions (known as the Directive health education approach).
- **The Informed Decision-Making Approach:** This involves providing individuals with information and skills for problem-solving and decision-making, enabling them to autonomously change their behaviors. This approach, also known as the non-directive health education approach, is commonly used in areas such as family planning methods. Health educators typically believe that it is preferable to help communities improve their problem-solving skills and provide them with information to support their decision-making process (Koelen & Ban, 2023). If there is a need to raise an alarm, such as during an epidemic, and specific behaviors need to be identified and encouraged, it may be justifiable to promote the adoption of certain behavior changes.

5.1.2. Targets in Health Education

Targets in health education encompass:

- Various individuals, such as specific clients utilizing particular services, specific patients, and individuals who are in good health.
- Groups such as students in a specific class or members of a youth group.
- Community such as a group of people who live in a particular village or area.

When choosing the scope of settings for health education interventions, they are typically described in relation to it. Settings are utilized to determine the appropriate resources and formal arrangements for implementing interventions, based on an understanding of their likely form (Koelen & Ban, 2023). Health education and promotion occur in various settings, including self-help groups, health facilities for patients, workplaces for employees, learning institutions for children, correction facilities for inmates, and refugee camps.

5.1.3. Who Bears the Responsibility for Health Education?

Health education is the responsibility of all individuals, as it is the process through which people improve, modify, or develop their health. It is also mandatory in any health and community development activities. These individuals primarily focus on collaborating with families and the local community to improve health and decrease the occurrence of diseases within their society through health education (Koelen & Ban, 2023).

The inference that can be made is that if health and other professionals do not actively participate in implementing health education in their daily work responsibilities, they are not fulfilling their obligations as required. When recommending a treatment, such as for skin infection or malaria, a healthcare professional should allocate sufficient time to elucidate the etiology of the illness and provide the client with detailed instructions on additional preventive measures to be followed. Merely relying on various medications is insufficient to effectively address the complications. As a result, individuals who lack health education may be more susceptible to the same disease and may not take the necessary precautions to prevent it. Healthcare professionals must also comprehend and embrace the fact that they serve as exemplars, imparting novel knowledge to the community.

5.1.4. The Responsibilities of a Health Educator

A health educator assists individuals in addressing and understanding the behavioral and causal factors contributing to their problems, as well as the process of resolving them.

- Achievements in discerning underlying behavioral motivations.
- Empowering individuals to comprehend the underlying factors behind their actions and health conditions.
- Encouraging people to generate their own solutions to the problems.
- Facilitating individuals in choosing the visual representation of their ideas, enabling them to identify the ones that are feasible to execute.
- Choosing an appropriate concept for a specific circumstance.

5.2. Interventions to Modify Behavior

Behavior, in this context, pertains to an action or activity that possesses a discernible frequency, duration, and purpose, which can be either intentional or reflexive. Our actions and behavior define us. Undoubtedly, professionalism is the essential element that binds and characterizes businesses and organizations as entities composed of individuals. Human health can transition from a state of wellness to a state of illness, often as a result of an individual's actions or inactions (Sheeran et al., 2017). Here are some instances illustrating how individuals' behaviors can impact their well-being:

- Utilizing preventive measures such as mosquito nets or insect sprays can effectively protect oneself from mosquitoes.

- Feeding children with a bottle increases their susceptibility to developing diarrhea.
- Engaging in unsafe sexual activities significantly raises the likelihood of experiencing unwanted pregnancies, contracting HIV/AIDS, and acquiring other sexually transmitted diseases.

Identifying the initiating factors, treating the disease, and preventing its occurrence are essential aspects of health education. This suggests that the actions, practices, and behaviors are all referring to the same concept.

5.2.1. Behaviors That Promote Good Health

These are measures that individuals in good health take to preserve their well-being. Examples of healthy behaviors include practicing good nutrition, engaging in breast feeding, and reducing health-damaging behaviors such as smoking.

- **Utilization Behavior:** Individuals showcase various elements of healthcare-seeking behavior, including antenatal care, child health, immunization, family planning, and other related services.
- **Compliance Behaviors:** These are determined by a range of distinctive traits, such as a track record of adhering to prescribed medications for conditions like tuberculosis.
- **Rehabilitation Behaviors:** These involve providing individuals with information about post-illness activities to prevent further disability.
- **Community Action:** This refers to the collective efforts of individuals, organizations, or communities to address changes and improvements in the environment in order to meet the specific needs of individuals facing particular challenges.

5.3. Factors That Influence Human Behavior

These are factors that make someone more likely to develop a certain condition. They include:

- **Knowledge:** Knowledge refers to the information that resides in the mind and has the potential to shape attitudes and values when combined with belief.
- **Enabling Factors:** These refer to various elements in the surroundings that support and facilitate favorable behaviors. They can include inherent, acquired elements, as well as any necessary actions or abilities to accomplish these behaviors (Sheeran et al., 2017). In order for motivation to work effectively, there are certain prerequisites that need to be in place. Enabling factors can be seen in the presence of organizational and liberal health resources. The government's policies and leadership in the health sector, along with their evident concern and support for it, are crucial factors to consider.
- **Reinforcing Factors:** These factors manifest subsequent to the behavior. Consistency in behavior over a prolonged period or the repetition of the same behavioral patterns can be highly beneficial. Reinforcing factors that play a crucial role

in influencing behavior include various individuals and entities. These include parents, siblings, close relatives, friends, teachers, classmates, employers, authorities, health officials, and leaders of society, as well as decision-makers.

5.4. Social Marketing in Health Promotion

As a means of influencing behavior, social marketing strives to assist individuals in achieving improved health, ultimately leading to a positive impact on the overall well-being of the population. The approach is primarily focused on proactively preventing potential output losses. One perspective is that it contradicts commercial health care marketing by focusing on reducing the need for cure-centric services (Lee & Kotler, 2015).

Health can be seen as a tangible market, where individuals invest social and monetary values and reap the benefits of health outputs from various products, services, or behaviors. By taking into account the principles and techniques that pertain to the wide realm of marketing, one can effectively sell the desired products, especially those related to health behaviors.

Social marketing can be described as the outcome of the progression in marketing development to a certain degree. This concept utilizes theories and strategies from the marketing discipline, such as:

- Exchange theory
- Customer-centric approach
- Competitor analysis
- Market research
- Studying customer behavior
- Identifying market areas
- Segmenting target audience
- Developing marketing mix strategies
- Planning, implementing, and evaluating marketing strategies

Through social marketing, the target community or intended consumers can experience a positive transformation, leading to social change (Lee & Kotler, 2015). This social behavioral change is in contrast to a concept that focuses on the behavior of the individual target audience rather than the behavior of a specific number of such audiences. In addition, social marketing aims to not only modify the behavior of the target audiences but also to sustain that behavior change among the audience. Some of the aspects of social marketing revolve around innovative and thought-provoking concepts.

There are notable distinctions between social concepts and tangible objects. To a certain degree, when it comes to intangible services, they fall into separate categories. The marketing subject is known for its abstract nature and the difficulty in pinpointing the exact characteristics of its purpose. This presents numerous challenges when it comes to promoting and conveying marketing messages, as it becomes unclear how to effectively reach the target audience (Lee & Kotler, 2015). Therefore, it is essential to develop a strategy for determining the key factors that contribute to the effectiveness of social marketing initiatives or a social marketing campaign.

5.4.1. Application of Social Marketing in Healthcare

Social marketing is comparable to traditional marketing as it employs strategies that can influence the behavior of a specific audience. Forward-thinking, savvy digital marketers have become adept at shaping consumers' decision-making and educating them about the advantages of taking a particular course of action, such as making a purchase. Nevertheless, various concepts and strategies for digital marketing can be applied to social marketing in healthcare. Some strategies that an organization may consider include blogging, search engine optimization, social marketing, and audience targeting. For example, a public health organization may find the following approach beneficial: in order to capture the audience's attention in today's saturated media landscape, it is crucial to utilize a variety of channels. Like any business, a public health organization must employ a variety of techniques to effectively influence decision-making in society. To achieve this, it is important to enhance the overall strategy that will help the marketing team stay focused on its mission and performance goals.

Before embarking on a social marketing campaign in healthcare, it is essential for an organization to carefully follow fundamental steps in its workflow (Figure 5.2).

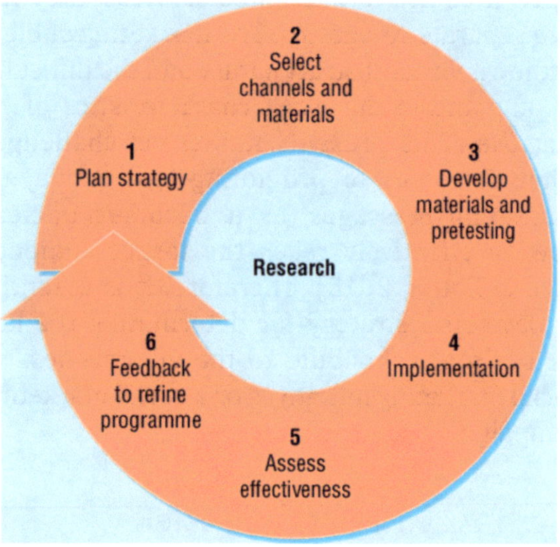

Figure 5.2. *How social marketing is used in healthcare.*

Source: Evans (2006).

- **Develop a Strategic Plan**: During the decision-making process in the strategic planning phase, the planners must define the goals, objectives, and mission statements of the social marketing campaign. They also need to determine the strategies that can be used to achieve these goals and objectives.
- **Choose Channels and Materials:** It is important for decision-makers to determine the channels they will utilize and the type of content they will include in their campaign, such as blogs or infographics, among other options.
- **Develop Additional Materials and Ideas and Assess the Approach:** Here, the organization will need to develop its marketing materials, test them in its target market, and refine them to increase the reach of its content.
- **Carry out the Program:** Once the content has been carefully prepared and refined, the public health entity can proceed with implementing the marketing strategy it has developed for all intended platforms.
- **Evaluate its Efficiency:** Given that the content is the primary message in a campaign, it is important for campaign managers to consistently monitor performance in order to assess the impact of the content.
- **Seek Input from Knowledgeable Individuals or Gather Feedback to Refine the Program:** Lastly, the marketing team will be tasked with evaluating the campaign's effectiveness, gathering any necessary information for refining the process, and beginning work on the next campaign.

5.5. Media Campaigns

Mass media campaigns utilize various methods to intervene and influence the behavior of entire population groups. Many targeting strategies aim to have a direct effect on the subject by stimulating either their cognitive or emotional functions. The design of these systems aims to shape human behavior at the individual level, particularly in the context of decision-making (Ahmad et al., 2016). The anticipated advantages involve removing or minimizing obstacles to change, promoting individuals to embrace change for better outcomes, and fostering a positive mindset towards change by associating it with positive experiences. These changes improve the rationale for transformation and offer a promising opportunity to develop new behaviors. For instance, an antismoking campaign could emphasize the drawbacks of smoking and the benefits of quitting. It might provide a support line for those seeking help, or remind smokers of the positive social expectations associated with quitting (Figure 5.3).

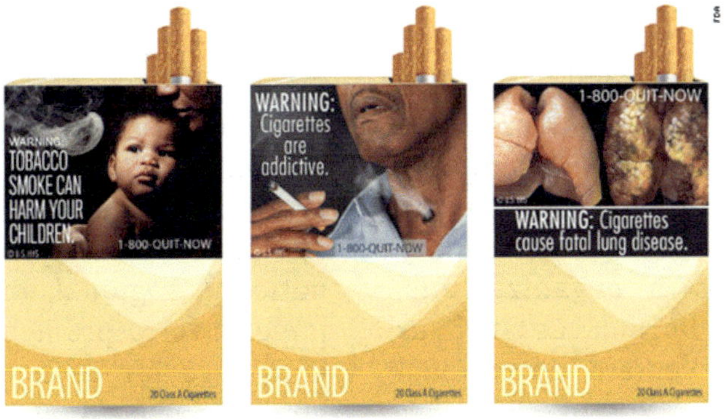

Figure 5.3. *Positive and instructive anti-smoking messages.*

Source: Cataldo et al. (2015).

Alternatively, it could connect quitting with positive self-images.

Some campaigns may incorporate elements of both approaches. It is also possible to bring about behavior change through alternative channels that can drive organizational change. There are multiple ways to approach organizational change based on this foundation. Mass media messages have the potential to stimulate and enhance discussions about health issues within an individual's communication network. These discussions, when reinforced personally, can lead to a greater depth and number of conversations, potentially influencing an individual's behavior. Furthermore, the dissemination of mass media messages to wide audiences has the power to shape collective behavior and influence individual decision-making, even without directly targeting individuals through knowledge or persuasion (Ahmad et al., 2016).

For example, after enjoying humorous television commercials that promote quitting smoking, a group of individuals may be inspired to create a club dedicated to assisting others in their journey to quit smoking. Imagine a situation where someone hasn't seen the television campaign, but then decides to support it and change their own behavior. Lastly, it is important to raise awareness about health issues and encourage public discussions that can influence government policies and bring about changes in people's behavior (Ahmad et al., 2016). For example, a campaign that aims to discourage smoking by highlighting the negative impact on non-smokers may not directly influence smokers' behavior. However, it can generate public support for a new policy that restricts smoking in certain areas. This policy could ultimately help resolve the issue as a whole and even motivate smokers to consider quitting for their own benefit.

5.6. Policy Development

Effective public policies have the power to improve the quality of life for individuals and communities, impacting their daily activities, education, employment, and even their dining experiences, all within their local surroundings. Policy development commonly takes place in various settings, including community organizations, non-profit organizations, and different types of workplaces such as health facilities, daycare centers, educational institutions, and industries (WHO 2020).

5.6.1. Actions for Health Promotion

5.6.1.1. Create a Strong Foundation for Effective Public Policy

The comprehension of health promotion extends beyond the purview of healthcare institutions. Health is a top priority for policy makers at every level. They are committed to considering the health implications of their actions and decisions, whether it's in the realm of policy, legislation, planning, implementation, or regulation. Health promotion policy is centered on various strategies and approaches including legislation, fiscal measures, taxation, and organizational changes. Collaborative efforts by policy-makers lead to enhanced health, income care, and social policies that promote fairness (WHO 2020). This effectively achieves the objective of creating safer and healthier products and services, promoting healthier public services, and creating better and cleaner environments for living, working, learning, and recreation. Health promotion policy must encourage and enable non-health sectors to identify obstacles to promoting healthy public policies and determine how to address or remove those obstacles. It is crucial that policy-makers prioritize making the healthier choice more accessible.

5.6.1.2. Foster Environments that Encourage Growth and Development

Our social structures are complex and interconnected. Wellbeing cannot be separated from various goals. The interdependent relationships between individuals and their current circumstances form the basis for a socioecological approach to health. The fundamental principle that underlies the global, national, regional, and local spheres is the imperative to promote equitable maintenance – to care for each other, our communities, and our shared environment (WHO 2020). It is imperative to highlight the preservation of natural resources worldwide as a global responsibility. Altering various aspects of life, such as work and recreation, can have a profound impact on one's overall well-being. Work and recreation should be a source of well-being for individuals. The way in which society organizes work should contribute to creating a healthy society. Wellbeing advancement creates living and working conditions that are safe, stimulating, fulfilling, and enjoyable.

An effective assessment of the impact of a rapidly changing climate, particularly in areas of innovation, work, energy production, and urbanization, is crucial and should be followed by action to ensure positive benefits to the well-being of the public (WHO 2020). The security and preservation of normal and constructed conditions and regular assets should be a top priority in any wellbeing advancement system.

5.6.1.3. Empower Community Initiatives

Wellbeing advancement focuses on practical community action to establish boundaries, determine strategies, and implement them in order to achieve improved health. Central to this interaction is the enhancement of networks – their ownership and management of their own endeavors and predetermined outcomes (WHO 2020). The local area's progress relies on utilizing the resources available to enhance personal growth and social support, as well as developing flexible systems to strengthen public involvement and direction in health-related issues. This necessitates complete and uninterrupted access to information, learning opportunities for health, as well as financial assistance.

5.6.1.4. Enhance Your Personal Skills

Wellbeing advancement supports personal and social development by providing information, education for health, and enhancing essential skills. By expanding the options available to individuals, they are empowered to have greater control over their own health and their environment, enabling them to make choices that promote well-being. It is crucial to empower individuals to continuously learn, prepare themselves for life's stages, and adapt to chronic illnesses and injuries (WHO 2020). This should be addressed in various settings such as school, home, work, and the local area. Activity is anticipated within educational, professional, commercial, and voluntary entities, as well as within the organizations themselves.

5.6.1.5. Revamp Health Services

The responsibility for promoting health in healthcare services is shared among individuals, local communities, healthcare professionals, healthcare institutions, and states. They should work together to develop a medical care framework that contributes to the pursuit of well-being. The role of the wellbeing area should evolve towards a more comprehensive approach to health promotion, going beyond its responsibility for providing clinical and therapeutic services. Wellbeing administrations should adopt a comprehensive approach that is sensitive to and respects social needs, as recommended by the World Health Organization in 2020. This order aims to address the needs of individuals and communities for an improved quality of life, while also fostering connections between the healthcare sector and broader social, political, economic, and environmental aspects. Shifting healthcare services also necessitates greater attention to health research as well as improvements in professional education and training. This should inspire a shift in attitude and approach to healthcare services that focuses on the holistic needs of the individual as a whole.

5.7. Environmental Change

The impacts of global environmental change on wellbeing vary from country to country. The disparity in the loss of life years between low pay African nations and Europe is expected to be significant. The fourth appraisal report of the Intergovernmental Board on Environmental Change suggests that low-income countries and vulnerable subpopulations are more likely to experience adverse health impacts (Fawzy et al., 2020). These variations are likely to increase in the future, not only due to differences in natural changes such as water shortages and soil erosion, but also because of disparities in economic conditions, social and human resources, political power, and local environmental dependence.

These differential wellbeing gambles also reflect the broader issue of access to global and local "public goods". A significant portion of the world's arable land has been taken over by private entities, leading to a decline in various wild species such as fish, animals, and plants. This unfortunate trend is exacerbated by population pressures and increased commercial activities. Additionally, the pricing of freshwater resources is increasingly being influenced by market forces (Fawzy et al., 2020). It is important for social arrangements to prioritize addressing the health disparities that arise from unequal access to environmental necessities. The accessibility of safe drinking water is a crucial issue that affects a significant portion of the global population. Approximately 1.1 billion people lack access to safe drinking water, while an even larger number, 2.6 billion individuals, do not have proper sanitation facilities. Water-related health risks can also arise from chemical contamination, such as arsenic, which can cause skin pigmentation, hyperkeratosis, cardiovascular disease, neuropathy, and cancer, in addition to past diarrheal infections.

Global environmental change caused by human activity is now widely acknowledged. Risks to overall health will arise through direct and indirect routes, and will mirror shifts in both natural environmental conditions and climate variation. The primary risks include:

- Effects of severe weather events such as hurricanes, floods, storms, and wildfires.
- Shifts in patterns of infectious diseases.
- Effects on crop production.
- Effects on freshwater resources.
- Disruption of ecosystems, such as wetlands acting as water filters.
- Displacement of vulnerable populations, such as those living in low-lying islands and coastal areas.
- Decrease in job opportunities.
- Severe weather events, illness, and poor health will disproportionately affect disadvantaged populations.

5.7.1. Ways for Health Professionals to Encourage Adaptive Strategies

Public education, particularly in healthcare settings like doctors' waiting rooms and hospital clinics

- Preventive programs such as vaccines, mosquito control, food hygiene and inspection, and nutritional supplementation
- Healthcare, specifically mental health and primary care, for communities facing environmental challenges
- Surveillance of disease, particularly infectious diseases, and important risk factors
- Predicting future health risks resulting from projected climate change
- Predicting future health risks and benefits from mitigation and adaptation strategies
- Training and professional development for the health sector workforce

5.7.2. Strategies That Go Beyond the Health Sector

- Developing frameworks to anticipate severe weather events such as heat waves and storms
- Implementing community support plans to protect vulnerable individuals
- Plan for sealed lodging in a controlled environment, prepare for urban living, implement water catchment systems, and adopt sustainable farming practices

- Preparedness for potential dangers, including the capacity of the healthcare system

While adaptive methodologies can help mitigate the effects of environmental change, a significant challenge in terms of public health is to halt the progression of climate change (Fawzy et al., 2020). This necessitates making strategic decisions at both public and global levels, involving significantly larger reductions in emissions than were proposed some years ago.

5.8. Community Mobilization

Local area preparation goes beyond mere motivation to participate in a specific health activity. The interconnectedness of various aspects allows for the local community's imagination to have an impact on the delivery of healthcare services. This impact can be seen in the physical, social, economic, and spiritual realms (Lydia, 2019). This impacts wellbeing frameworks and therefore, it is evident that the community should be involved in all aspects of healthcare, considering its significant potential.

The local area's contribution is a reflection of their sense of responsibility and ownership. It demonstrates the local area's ability to make decisions regarding its projects. The components of local area contribution encompass all the achievements pursued in the decision-making regarding governance, organization, resources, economics, and distribution of health for-all initiatives.

It is crucial that the three terms – association, activation, and association – are commonly used interchangeably to refer to the entire continuum (Lydia, 2019). It is evident that each individual within the community has a profound impact on the other members, resulting in a complex web of interconnectedness.

5.8.1. Key Aspects of Community Mobilization

Local area assembly is often seen as a means of achieving the predetermined goals of health initiatives or services. From this perspective, local area preparation is seen as a temporary endeavor that is influenced by the resources, time, and location at hand. The local area needs to focus on setting targets, developing systems, considering functional viewpoints, allocating resources, and conducting evaluations. It is a job that requires a more hands-off approach, focusing on the conceptual aspects rather than the practical execution of predetermined tasks (Lydia, 2019).

This is an example of the application of community training as a strategy and, in essence, community training is spontaneous and temporary. On the other hand, the process of preparing individuals can be seen as a way to empower the community and enhance its capacity to make informed decisions and effectively manage various aspects of its development, such as planning, implementation, and progress in all areas that impact its quality of life. This latest model aligns with the concept of collective assistance, where all employees are expected to be accountable to the public they serve.

5.8.2. The Purpose of Community Mobilization

Development and health: It is now more evident than ever that improving health status begins in spaces that exist outside the hierarchical structure of the health services. Enhancement of overall well-being is influenced by various factors, but particularly by the community (Lydia, 2019). Addressing neediness, a crucial factor impacting well-being, requires the implementation of long-term and medium-term development approaches.

- **Empowering Individuals to Become Self-Sufficient:** Wellbeing is a crucial factor in determining one's quality of life. People are the primary assets in the pursuit of achieving improved health for themselves. Notable achievements in improving health are made when simple and effective measures, such as oral rehydration therapy, are introduced because individuals are actively involved in their own care. The role of networks in the healthcare sector should be evaluated to enhance community management of health programs. Community preparation is all about helping individuals help themselves.
- **The Establishment of a Robust Primary Healthcare Infrastructure:** The scope of enhancing essential medical services is vast and intricate, extending beyond the clinical field to involve various other partners whose potential should be wisely utilized to achieve sustainable health for all. Essential medical care addresses a wide range of factors that impact health, such as poverty, lack of education (especially among women), population growth, unemployment, rural to urban migration, substance abuse, environmental issues, and epidemics. Current medical care systems fail to take into account these factors that influence health and therefore need to be reoriented.

Local community involvement plays a crucial role in ensuring the effectiveness of the healthcare system in addressing the factors at hand (Lydia, 2019). When individuals prioritize thorough preparation, the fundamental healthcare system will become fair, sustainable, adequate, continuous, and uncomplicated.

- **Promoting and Safeguarding Health:** Wellbeing is a fundamental right and a responsibility that the community should contribute to. Given the current state of affairs and the shifting patterns in public health, it is crucial for individuals to prioritize their well-being and safety, and to actively pursue a healthy lifestyle. The knowledge gained from participating in illness prevention projects should be expanded to address the growing burden of noncommunicable diseases, drug abuse and addiction, alcoholism, promiscuity, violence, and accidents. This highlights the significant strengths in understanding the causes and implementing effective strategies to combat the emerging threats posed by these new diseases.

5.9. Health Coaching

A health and wellness coach can support individuals in optimizing their lives, regardless of any chronic medical conditions they may have. Similarly, a sports coach can aid athletes in honing their skills and achieving excellence in their chosen sport. Although the coaching process shares similarities with talk therapy, it distinguishes itself by allowing the individual receiving coaching to establish their own objectives and devise strategies to achieve them (Figure 5.4).

For individuals seeking support in various health challenges like weight loss, stress management, chronic disease management, nutrition and exercise improvement, smoking cessation, addiction recovery, and adapting to life-changing health events like a heart attack, health coaches are frequently sought after (Dimitrov, 2016). Although there are certain similarities between the work of a life coach and a health coach, the scope of a life coach is much broader, encompassing executive coaching, job challenges, and professional effectiveness.

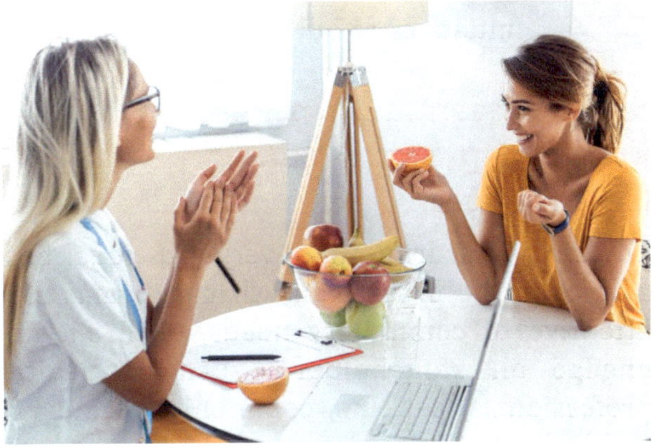

Figure 5.4. *Health and wellness coach.*

Source: Health & Wellness Coaches | VA West Palm Beach Health Care | Veterans Affairs (2024).

Motivational interviewing is a vital coaching technique where a coach utilizes open-ended questions to assist their client in discovering their own motivations for desiring change. Instead of simply being told to lose weight, a coach might ask you to imagine how your life could change if you were able to shed the weight you've been struggling with. Individuals who undergo personal transformations based on their own motivations and preferences are more likely to achieve success compared to those who are directed by others (Dimitrov, 2016). The latter is less inspiring and is more likely to create a reluctance to embrace change. This idea has been proven to be effective in numerous research studies. Coaching philosophy emphasizes finding effective strategies that can improve your situation, while traditional psychology has traditionally focused on identifying problems and seeking solutions. This implies that a coach will collaborate with you to utilize your strengths in order to enhance the health habits you want to address, instead of actively seeking out problems to concentrate on (Dimitrov, 2016).

5.10. Evaluation and Monitoring in Health Promotion

In the healthcare industry, monitoring and evaluation (M&E) is an essential procedure that ensures healthcare interventions and programs are effective, successful, and responsive to community needs.

5.10.1. Importance of M&E in the Health Sector

Understanding and implementing monitoring and evaluation is crucial for improving the quality and effectiveness of healthcare initiatives and services. Furthermore, it provides valuable data that can inform evidence-based decisions regarding resource allocation, intervention design, and healthcare outcome improvement. It also helps in identifying the strengths and weaknesses of healthcare delivery systems (McKenzie et al., 2022). M&E can also enhance transparency and accountability in the healthcare industry by providing data on the effectiveness of healthcare systems and providers. M&E can also contribute to ensuring that healthcare services and initiatives prioritize human rights and dignity, while also being responsive to the needs of the community. M&E can play a crucial role in ensuring that healthcare programs and services are developed with a strong focus on the needs and preferences of the community. This can be achieved by actively involving stakeholders, including patients, healthcare practitioners, and community members, in the design and implementation of M&E systems.

5.10.2. Essential Elements of an M&E System in the Health Sector

A comprehensive M&E system in the health sector should encompass the following components:

- **Clearly Defined Indicators and Objectives:** It is crucial to establish measurable and achievable indicators and objectives as the basis for monitoring and evaluation. Collaboratively with stakeholders, it is important to establish objectives and indicators that align with the overall goals of the healthcare program or service.
- **Data Collection:** M&E in the health sector requires the systematic gathering of data using appropriate instruments and techniques (McKenzie et al., 2022). This involves identifying the most appropriate data sources, such as medical records, questionnaires, and interviews, and ensuring that data is collected in a consistent and standardized manner.
- **Data Analysis:** Once collected, data needs to be carefully and systematically analyzed. This involves analyzing the data using the appropriate statistical techniques and tools and ensuring that the results are precise and reliable.
- **Reporting and Feedback:** It is crucial to efficiently and expeditiously communicate M&E findings with stakeholders. This involves generating reports that are clear and comprehensible, and providing stakeholders with the opportunity to contribute to the M&E's findings.
- **Application of Results:** In order to improve healthcare outcomes and inform decision-making, it is important to utilize the findings from monitoring and evaluation. This involves identifying areas that require improvement based on the results and developing plans and initiatives to address them.

5.10.3. Essential Principles for Monitoring and Evaluation in the Health Sector

Inclusivity: Ensuring that every individual has a voice in the process and that programs are attentive to community needs, M&E should engage all stakeholders, such as health professionals, patients, community members, and legislators.

- **Clear Objectives:** M&E should have clear and well-defined goals that align with the objectives of any health program or intervention. The SMART framework is essential for developing objectives. It ensures that objectives are specific, measurable, achievable, relevant, and time-bound.
- **Utilization of Appropriate Techniques:** Depending on the nature of the program or intervention being evaluated, M&E should employ suitable methods and tools to collect data. These techniques should be reliable, credible, and appropriate for the local culture.
- **Data Quality:** Ensuring the quality of M&E data is crucial, with a focus on timeliness, accuracy, and reliability. For effective trend

analysis and comparisons, it is crucial to collect data consistently over time.

- **Ethical Considerations:** M&E should be conducted with a strong sense of morality and responsibility, ensuring that moral principles are upheld and participants' privacy and confidentiality are protected.
- **Adaptability:** M&E should be able to adjust to evolving circumstances. The outcomes of monitoring and evaluation may necessitate adjustments to programs and interventions to ensure their relevance and effectiveness.
- **Application of Findings**: The results of M&E should guide decision-making and program enhancements. Stakeholders should be provided with M&E reports that are presented in a concise and easily understandable manner, accompanied by actionable recommendations (McKenzie et al., 2022).
- **Ensuring Longevity:** Incorporating monitoring and evaluation (M&E) from the outset is crucial for the sustained success of a health program or intervention (McKenzie et al., 2022). It is essential for program budgets and planning procedures to include monitoring and evaluation (M&E) to ensure adequate funding.

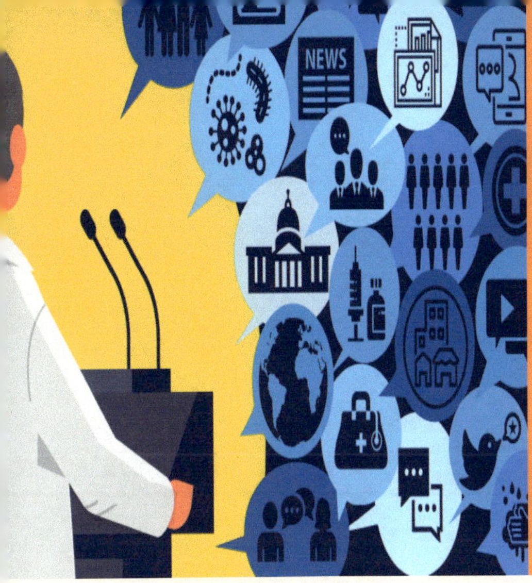

Chapter 6

HEALTH COMMUNICATION IN HEALTH PROMOTION

Contents

The interaction between the patient and the healthcare practitioner can greatly benefit from clear and efficient communication in various ways. Individuals may choose to embrace proactive wellness and health practices when they possess a greater understanding of their own well-being (Rimal & Lapinski, 2009). In addition, it can help patients develop a comprehensive understanding of the current methods used to manage their health, particularly in emergency medical situations. Furthermore, effective communication has the potential to cultivate a sense of trust between the patient and the practitioner, thereby enhancing a patient's willingness to follow the advice provided. These components offer numerous long-term benefits, such as reducing patient visits, lowering costs, and improving patient outcomes (Figure 6.1).

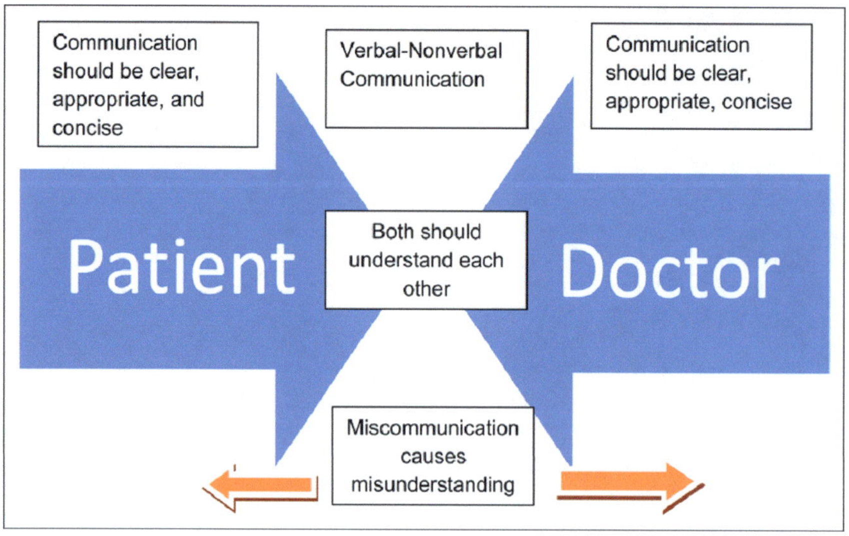

Figure 6.1. *Effective communication in health care.*

Source: Ellahham (2021).

In the healthcare industry, effective communication is increasingly important due to the rising use of technology. It can reduce the likelihood of patients making poor or inaccurate decisions about their health due to misinformation. In addition, it can enhance communication among various medical professionals who may need to collaborate on patient care across multiple locations. In addition, this could potentially increase the likelihood of being able to offer quality care.

6.1. Forms of Communication in Health Care

There are numerous communication channels available in the current healthcare environment to assist doctors in staying informed about the latest developments.

- **Patient Portals:** Medical facilities have the ability to develop patient portals, providing individuals with the opportunity to register and gain exclusive access to their personal health records. Relevant educational health material tailored to the patient's specific needs can be shared on the patient portal. It is indeed feasible to provide access to clinical summaries. These summaries may provide a recap of the patient's most recent visit or an explanation of the results of any recent tests, as discussed by Rimal and Lapinski in 2009. It may be beneficial to include suggestions, such as the need for follow-up appointments, in the summary as well.
- **Emailing:** Medical professionals have realized the significance of addressing patient inquiries through email rather than taking phone calls. Emails serve as useful reminders for submitting orders to other providers or addressing common inquiries efficiently. Using emails instead of phone calls for medication requests is a more efficient approach as it helps save time.

- **Texting:** Prescription reminders, patient portal notifications, and appointment delays can all be efficiently communicated through texting, ensuring prompt and convenient updates (Rimal & Lapinski, 2009). Playing a vital role in patient security measures such as two-factor login authentication, it can also contribute to the maintenance of the security of a patient's portal information.
- **Social Media:** Utilizing social media is a cost-effective way to effectively communicate with a large audience. We can provide responses to general inquiries and offer information. Responding to critical remarks posted on social media can potentially alter the public's perception of your medical center (Rimal & Lapinski, 2009). In addition, the hospital can promote specific health-related events. Sharing accurate and reliable information during public health emergencies is crucial in preventing panic and the spread of misinformation.
- **Apps and Websites:** Applications can be utilized by healthcare providers to effectively reach and engage with diverse populations. For those with a thirst for knowledge, they may consider creating a website filled with informative health facts. They could also offer video footage of real patients to illustrate how a treatment works.

  A potential development by healthcare providers could be an app that prompts users to maintain certain healthy habits, such as exercise or monitoring their blood sugar levels (Rimal & Lapinski, 2009). Patients facing similar challenges can also support each other through online communities. Patients may also have the option to engage in live chat.

6.2. Theories of Communication

An essential aspect of human interaction is communication. Effective communication is crucial for conveying ideas, establishing relationships, and fostering comprehension in various settings—whether personal, professional, or societal. The art of communication is enriched by a multitude of ideas, which allow us to delve into its intricate nature (Golding & Murdock, 1978). Acquiring knowledge about these theories will enhance your communication skills and provide valuable insights into the exchange, interpretation, and assimilation of information.

6.2.1. Transmission Model of Communication

The transmission model of communication is a fundamental theory in the field that helps to elucidate the key elements of communication.

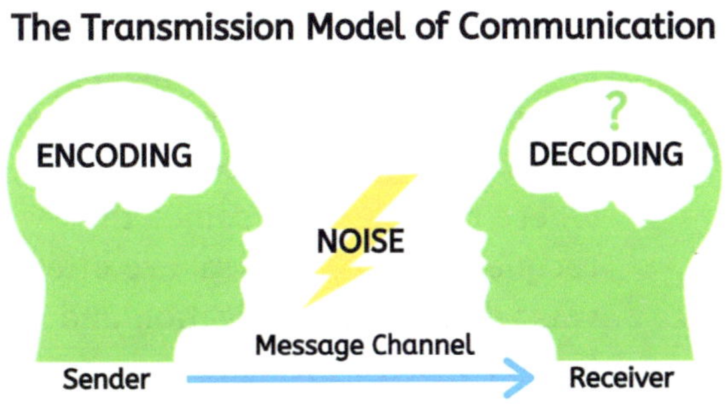

Figure 6.2. *Transmission model of communication.*

Source: Lapum et al. (2020).

Based on this model, communication is seen as a linear process that includes a sender, a recipient, and a message. The process of communication involves the sender encoding the message, transmitting it through a channel, and the recipient decoding it. This approach prioritizes the importance of precision and lucidity in conveying information (Figure 6.2). In the transmission model, the sender converts the message, turning ideas and thoughts into a format that can be transmitted to the recipient. Encoding involves carefully selecting words, strategically organizing thoughts, and considering nonverbal cues. Once the message has been encoded, it is then transmitted through various channels such as written text, spoken communication, or digital media (Golding & Murdock, 1978). Later on, the recipient deciphers the communication and applies their own context and understanding to the sent data. This process of sending and receiving demonstrates the intricate dynamics of communication and highlights the significance of accurate decoding and clear encoding for the effective transfer of messages.

- **Limitations and Criticisms of the Transmission Model:** While the transmission model provides a basic understanding of communication, it is important to acknowledge its limitations and criticisms. Skeptics argue that by portraying communication as a linear, one-way process, this model oversimplifies the complex nature of communication. Feedback loops, where the sender becomes the recipient and vice versa, are often what define communication and lead to a more dynamic and engaged discussion (Golding & Murdock, 1978). In addition, the transmission model fails to consider the impact of context, cultural variations, and individual interpretations on communication. By recognizing these limitations, we can expand our understanding of communication and seek out more comprehensive theories that account for the intricate dynamics of interpersonal connections.

6.2.2. Social Learning Theory of Communication

The social learning theory of communication delves into the ways in which our communication actions and skills are influenced by observational learning. Based on this thesis (initially proposed by Albert Bandura) individuals acquire and enhance their communication abilities through observation, imitation, and emulation of others. Aside from observing individuals in our immediate environment, media depictions also educate us on social interactions.

6.2.2.1. The Impact of Social Reinforcement

The social learning theory suggests that social reinforcement plays a significant role in shaping our communication choices. Embracing effective communication techniques is highly encouraged through positive reinforcement, while discouraging improper or inefficient behavior through negative reinforcement. This implies that we can enhance our own skills and encourage positive social interactions by observing and emulating individuals who employ influential, polite, and articulate communication (Golding & Murdock, 1978). However, by consciously steering clear of and distancing ourselves from unproductive communication models, we can better navigate away from ineffective communication practices.

Positive role models can serve as sources of inspiration and provide examples of effective communication strategies. They can be found in a wide range of environments, such as professional settings, interpersonal connections, and public speaking engagements. We can gain valuable insights from their successful tactics and incorporate them into our own communication styles, enhancing our ability to effectively convey ideas and foster understanding.

Engaging in the learning process and being mindful are crucial for applying the social learning theory of communication. Recognizing the significance of social reinforcement enables us to evaluate the communication and behavior choices we make for ourselves (Golding & Murdock, 1978). We can identify areas that require improvement and actively strive to implement more effective communication techniques by engaging in self-reflection and assessment. This involves consciously selecting inspiring individuals to emulate, seeking and accepting feedback from others, and actively refining our ability to communicate in different situations.

The social learning theory of communication highlights the significance of observational learning in shaping our communication abilities. By actively engaging in the learning process, closely observing and emulating successful communication habits, and seeking out positive role models, we can enhance our ability to communicate effectively, build rapport, and foster understanding in various situations. Embracing this principle empowers us to select our words thoughtfully, leading to more profound and fruitful relationships with others.

6.2.3. Coordinated Management of Meaning (CMM)

The coordinated management of meaning (CMM) theory, developed by Golding and Murdock in 1978, delves into the intricate process of meaning production in communication. This concept suggests that effective communication involves the collaborative construction and exploration of shared understandings, rather than just the transmission of facts. Understanding that social roles, cultural norms, and situational dynamics all play a crucial role in communication, CMM highlights the importance of context in shaping meaning (Figure 6.3).

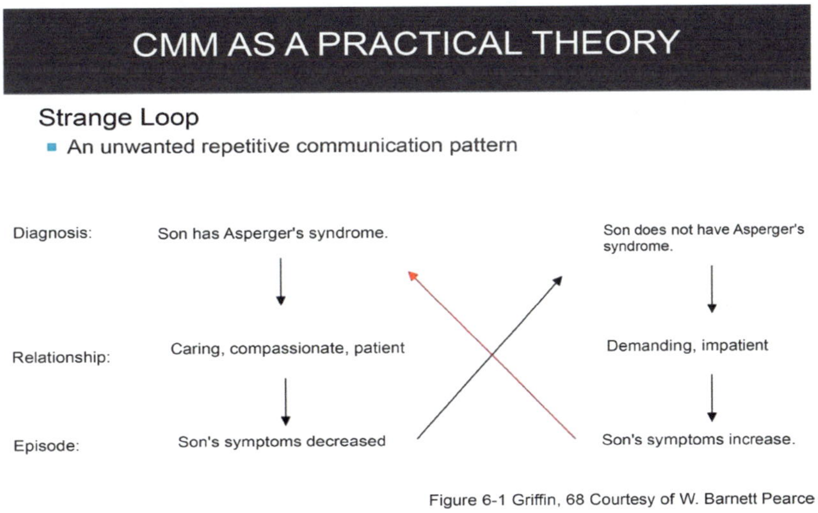

Figure 6.3. *Coordinated management of meaning.*

Source: Akina (2013).

An appreciation for context as a guiding principle in communication is essential to the CMM philosophy. The context encompasses the broader social and cultural factors that influence how we understand and interpret communications. By considering the context of communication, we can gain a deeper understanding of the intricate layers of meaning embedded in our relationships. This heightened awareness enables us to navigate diverse cultural settings, adapt our communication approach accordingly, and foster deeper understanding and fruitful collaborations. CMM highlights the importance of communication in shaping shared realities in a dynamic manner. Through their interactions, individuals collaboratively develop interpretations and understanding by consistently negotiating and coordinating meaning. This concept emphasizes the deliberate construction of meanings through social interaction, rather than assuming that meanings are inherent in words or messages (Golding & Murdock, 1978). We can approach communication with a mindset of receptiveness, inquisitiveness, and preparedness to understand different perspectives if we recognize the collaborative nature of constructing meaning. Interpretation plays a crucial role in the CMM framework. Individuals mold the significance they derive from messages through the application of their own cultural perspectives, personal interpretations, and life experiences to the process of communication. This philosophy highlights the importance of embracing and recognizing diverse interpretations, while engaging in discussions to clarify and reconcile conflicting perspectives. We can foster a shared understanding by encouraging respectful and transparent dialog, allowing us to bridge gaps in perspectives and reach common ground.

6.3. Audience Segmentation

One of the main objectives of audience segmentation is to enhance communication effectiveness and establish stronger connections by identifying distinct subgroups within the target population. Segmentation is the process of identifying groups of individuals who share similar needs and interests in relation to the behavior you want to modify (Peterson, 1992).

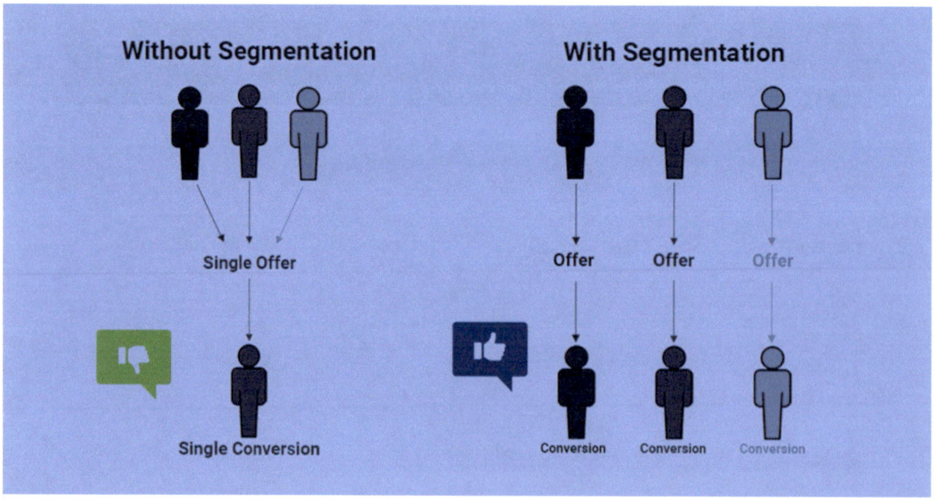

Figure 6.4. *Audience segmentation.*

Source: Admin (2023).

When group members possess similar traits, they tend to respond to SBCC activities in a similar manner. Additionally, this allows you to concentrate on the specific groups that would derive the greatest advantage from the program. It guarantees that the activities you select are the most suitable and impactful for the intended audiences, and aids in the development of tailored messages and materials (Figure 6.4). The main findings obtained from the situation analysis should address the question of which individuals' behavior needs to be modified in order to bring about a change in the health situation. Understanding audience segmentation is crucial at this stage.

Primary audiences are the crucial individuals to target with messaging. It is important to focus on practicing the desired behavior with these individuals, as they are the ones who may experience the immediate impact. On the other hand, they could be the individuals entrusted with the responsibility of making decisions on behalf of those who would benefit from the actions. According to Peterson (1992), sub-audiences can be created by dividing primary audiences into smaller segments. For instance, the primary audience for nursing is typically pregnant women and mothers of young children. Influential audiences are individuals who possess the ability to shape or guide the actions of the primary audience. Examples of influential audiences include families and community members, as well as individuals who shape societal norms, influence laws, or change public perceptions of the activity. It is crucial to prioritize the influence of setting.

6.3.1. Developing Audience Profiles

Developing an audience profile is an essential task in understanding the individuals who will be engaging with your content. These profiles bring each audience segment to life and guide the development of communication messaging and activity planning. It is important for the profile to accurately capture the characteristics of the target audience and effectively portray an individual within that group who can serve as a representative (Peterson, 1992). When decisions are made with consideration for the potential impact on individuals, a greater understanding of the target audience can be achieved. This, in turn, allows for more precise and effective communication strategies.

It would be advisable to conduct additional research in order to address any discrepancies in the information provided by the situation analysis regarding the accuracy of audience segments. For example, conducting formative research on provider attitudes and other factors that impact their behavior, such as policies, training, supervision, or resources, can be extremely important for all audiences of health providers. This data can be used to enhance the strategy and better understand the audience profile.

6.4. Developing the Message

Health communicators are influenced by health communication, which empowers them to have an impact on both public and individual literacy. Crafting persuasive health communication messages can be a challenging task, regardless of the desired change in consumer behavior. Changing your behavior can be quite challenging, as demonstrated by the research conducted by Head, et al., in 2013. In order to bring about social change and alter people's attitudes, it is crucial for qualified communicators to create and distribute authoritative and clear messages on subjects pertaining to public and individual health.

Whether messages about health are effective or not can vary. An idea that can be utilized to elucidate effective message designs is McGuire's hierarchy. McGuire emphasizes the importance of several key steps that viewers should take before acting.

- It is crucial to pay close attention to the message at hand.
- Viewers should take care to nurture their interest in the message, ensuring that it remains a priority.
- It is essential to recognize the message for what it is, acknowledging its significance.
- Viewers should carefully consider the message, taking into account its implications and potential impact.
- Enhance your skills in the relevant areas.
- Embrace the perspective conveyed in the message (change in attitude).
- Remember the message.
- Remember to retrieve the message from memory when it is applicable.
- Make a deliberate decision to take action based on the information.

Successfully completing each of these steps relies on a set of communication variables:

- The source of the communication should be credible and appealing.
- The design of the message, including its structure and style, is an important aspect to consider.
- The channel's features, including its directness, are worth noting.
- When considering the recipient of the communication, it is important to take into account their qualities, such as their disposition and level of education.

Health messages play a crucial role in determining whether behavior change efforts are successful or not. By focusing on various communication variables and their impact on different phases, we can better understand how to effectively convey important information (Head et al., 2013). The ease of completing one step may be inversely proportional to the difficulty of the next step. Effective communication requires finding a balance between captivating content and ensuring clarity for the audience. In addition, it is important to note that even when working towards similar goals, different audiences may require different forms of communication.

When crafting a persuasive message, it is important to consider the following:

- The message will captivate and maintain the audience's attention.
- The most crucial points of the message are presented initially.
- The meaning is clearly apparent.
- Asking the audience to complete a task that is relatively straightforward.
- The message effectively utilizes incentives.
- A comprehensive analysis is provided, highlighting both the benefits and potential drawbacks.
- The messenger is widely recognized as a trustworthy and dependable source of information.
- The messages are coherent and logical.
- The message is well-suited for the target demographic.

6.5. Channels of Communication

A communication channel is the method through which a message is transmitted to its intended recipient. There are three main channels through which information can be conveyed: oral, written (in hard copy print or digital versions), and electronic and multimedia (Ahlsvvede, 1971). Interpersonal channels such as in-person meetings, home visits, training sessions, group discussions, and counseling, have proven to be highly effective in imparting complex skills that require two-way communication between patients and healthcare providers. These methods further enhance the credibility of messages.

6.5.1. Interpersonal Channels

Interpersonal channels are often considered the most effective for sharing information, teaching intricate skills that involve interaction between patients and healthcare professionals, and establishing credibility for messages. The channels for communication include various methods such as face-to-face communication, home visits, training, group discussions, and counseling.

6.5.2. Broadcast Channels

This is another effective way to reach a large audience. A good example is the use of radio and television, which have the advantage of quickly and frequently reaching a significant portion of the target population. Print media, such as fliers, posters, and booklets, are widely regarded as highly effective in promptly reinforcing important communication points.

When choosing channels for communicating health message, it is important to remember the following:

- Having the correct products, audience, and health message is of utmost importance.
- Equally important is considering how to effectively convey them through efficient means.
- Select channels that are appropriate for the target audience and readily available. For instance, it is important to schedule radio messages during times when the target audience is most likely to be listening. This ensures that the messages reach the intended audience effectively.
- Print materials are best suited for individuals who possess a certain level of literacy and are accustomed to acquiring knowledge through written and visual resources. It is important to ensure that materials are distributed in highly visible and easily accessible locations that are commonly visited by the target audience.
- It is important to remember that each channel serves a specific purpose. Using multiple channels simultaneously can be highly advantageous. Using multiple channels can enhance the reach, frequency, and effectiveness of communication messages. The concept of "media mix" often pertains to the organization of these various channels.

According to Ahlsvvede (1971), when a message is returned with comments from the recipient to the sender, it is considered to have received feedback. It is important for the sender to ascertain whether the recipient has comprehended and acted upon the messages, as well as the level of reception they have received. The communication process is concluded. Feedback has the power to bring about a significant transformation in the knowledge, attitude, practice, and behavior of the person receiving it. When an intended change in knowledge, attitude, or practice occurs, it can have a positive impact. However, if the change does not take place, it can have a negative effect.

6.6. Health Literacy

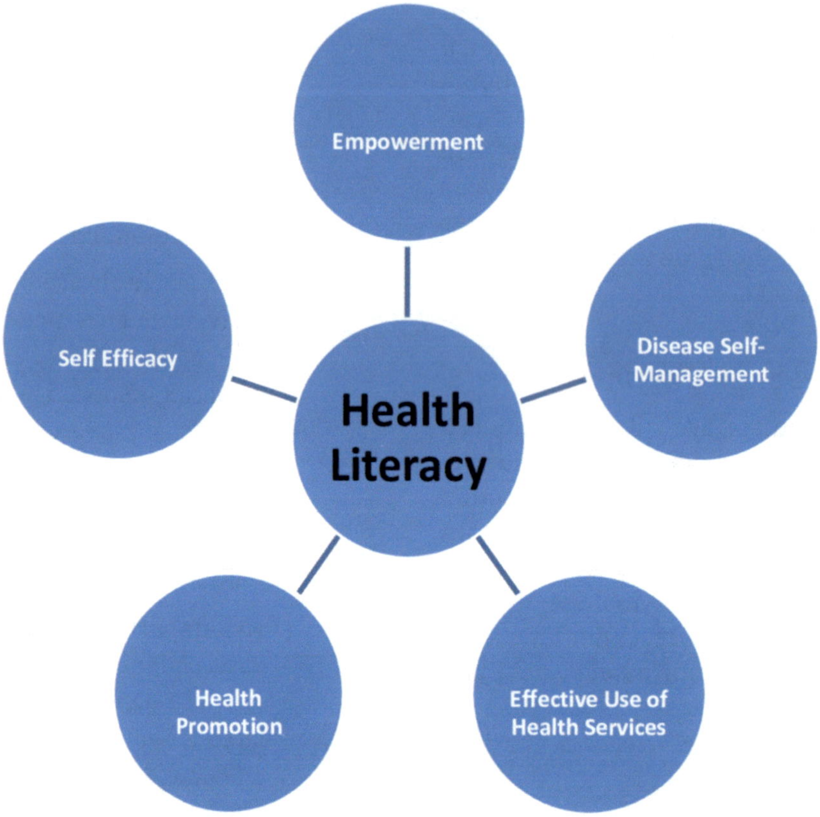

Figure 6.5. *Health literacy – a personal strategy for patients.*

Source: Doyle et al. (2012).

Personal health literacy refers to the skill of finding, understanding, and using resources and information to make informed decisions about health for oneself and others (Andrus & Roth, 2002) (Figure 6.5).

Organizational health literacy refers to the level at which organizations effectively support individuals in finding, understanding, and using resources and information to make informed decisions and take appropriate actions regarding their health and the health of others.

It is essential for individuals to possess the ability to find, understand, and utilize health resources at various points in their lives. This emphasizes the significance of health literacy. It is crucial to prioritize our health every day, rather than solely relying on medical professionals and facilities. Understanding health literacy is crucial for safeguarding our well-being, proactively addressing health concerns, and efficiently handling any preexisting conditions. Health literacy issues can occur even for individuals who possess strong reading skills and are comfortable with numbers when they lack comprehension of medical terminology or knowledge about their own bodily functions.

It is crucial for individuals to carefully evaluate the potential risks and benefits that can have an impact on their overall safety and well-being. Additionally, they should possess the ability to accurately interpret statistical data in order to make informed decisions.

One common problem in health literacy occurs when people or groups create health information that is overly complicated and then share it with others. When individuals are faced with the challenge of navigating health services that involve numerous unfamiliar, unclear, or even contradicting steps, it can inadvertently contribute to a problem with health literacy.

As a health literacy ambassador, it is crucial for you to emphasize the importance of utilizing health literacy principles to top management, employees, colleagues, and community leaders (Andrus & Roth, 2002).

6.6.1. Why It Is Important to Create a Health-Literate Workplace

Here are some key points to consider:

Ensure that the topics you discuss are relevant. When health information is written in complex language, it can be challenging for most people to understand and use. Poor health literacy has a significant impact on both the health outcomes and financial burden of the healthcare system. By enhancing health literacy, we have the potential to achieve significant cost savings of more than $25 billion each year and prevent nearly 1 million hospital admissions.

By implementing various communication strategies and techniques, we can improve health literacy. Clear communication involves effectively presenting familiar ideas, phrases, figures, and graphics in a manner that resonates with the intended audience.

Prior to releasing any material to the public, it is crucial to thoroughly test it and actively seek feedback. Having the trust and confidence of your audience is crucial in order for them to value and follow your advice. Language can be exclusionary, as it has the power to leave certain individuals out. Health fairness is promoted through transparency in communication.

Clear communication is essential for streamlining the translation process. It suggests that you have the ability to effectively and efficiently communicate with both readers and non-native English speakers.

6.7. Cultural Competence in Health Promotion

There are various factors that can shape a person's values, beliefs, and behaviors regarding health and well-being. These factors encompass a wide range of aspects, such as race, ethnicity, nationality, language, gender, financial class, physical and mental ability, sexual orientation, and occupation. Understanding and integrating these variables into the delivery and structure of the healthcare system is referred to as cultural competency in the field of medicine (Chiu, 2009). The goal of culturally competent health care services is to provide the best care to all patients, regardless of their color, ethnicity, cultural background, level of literacy in English, or other factors.

Here are some common strategies to improve communication between patients and healthcare providers and implement systemic changes in the healthcare industry:

- Provide assistance with interpreting.
- Attract and retain a diverse workforce.
- Provide guidance to enhance knowledge, skills, and cultural awareness.
- Collaborate with traditional healers.

- Utilize the expertise of community health professionals.
- One important aspect to consider when developing health promotion materials is the inclusion of attitudes and values that are specific to a particular culture.
- Ensure that the materials resonate with the target audience and effectively communicate the intended messages.
- Engage community and family members in the decision-making process regarding healthcare.
- Strategically place clinics in easily accessible locations to ensure that specific individuals can conveniently reach them.
- Consider extending the hours of operation.
- Have multilingual staff available at the appointment desk, help lines, and for handling medical bills and other written documents, in addition to the clinical setting.

It is imperative for health personnel to undergo training in culturally competent service delivery to enhance the system's level of cultural competence. It is worth noting that numerous training programs have been developed across the country. However, there has been a lack of consistency and integration in incorporating these initiatives into the education of healthcare professionals (Chiu, 2009). It is important to keep in mind that the development of cultural competence is an ongoing process that builds upon previous knowledge and experience.

Being well-versed in every culture can be quite challenging. Therefore, it is important to consider that training methods focused solely on information have their limitations and are most effective when combined with methods that teach more transferable skills. As an example, individuals can utilize skills such as effective communication and comprehensive medical history-taking techniques when working with a diverse clientele (Chiu, 2009). Having a curious mindset, showing empathy, demonstrating respect, and maintaining humility can greatly enhance the clinical interaction and offer valuable insights into the patient's personal preferences and perspectives. Understanding that culture is just one factor that shapes an individual's health beliefs and actions requires a method that emphasizes investigation, contemplation, and examination throughout the process of providing care.

6.7.1. Professional Guidelines that Promote Cultural Competence

Professional associations representing a variety of health professionals, such as doctors, psychologists, social workers, family medicine physicians, and pediatricians, have made significant contributions to the development of culturally competent practices. This can be achieved through legislation, studies, and educational initiatives. The American Medical Association provides a wide range of resources and information on various aspects of the medical field. These include state medical societies, physician associations, medical specialty groups, publications, curriculum, training materials, and other activities. Many organizations have established policies regarding cultural competence for their members. One example is the Society of Teachers of Family Medicine, which has developed a set of criteria for curriculum materials aimed at teaching cultural sensitivity and competency to family medicine residents and other health professionals. This initiative is the result of ten years of dedicated work (Chiu, 2009). The instructions for improving attitudes focus on the following areas:

- Understanding the impact of sociocultural elements on patients, doctors, and the therapeutic alliance.

- Recognizing the importance of doctors understanding the cultural aspects of health and illness.
- Showing a willingness to make healthcare more accessible for patients.
- Being aware of personal biases towards individuals from different cultures.
- Valuing and respecting cultural diversity.
- Recognizing the responsibility to combat prejudice and discrimination such as racism, classism, ageism, sexism, homophobia, and other forms of bigotry in healthcare settings.

Health care providers and systems are increasingly recognizing the importance of cultural competence. Health systems are increasingly adopting comprehensive plans to address the needs of racial and ethnic minorities. This is driven by a multitude of factors. One important factor to consider is the increasing number of state and federal regulations that are pushing health systems to become more attentive to the ever-growing diversity of the population. In addition, it is worth noting that the attainment of the federal government's Healthy People 2010 goal of eliminating health disparities among different racial and ethnic groups can be seen as closely linked to these endeavors (Chiu, 2009).

Furthermore, many health systems have recognized the strategic advantage of implementing cultural competence initiatives. These initiatives aim to increase the engagement and participation of racial and ethnic minority communities in their health plans – benefiting both consumers and providers. It is important to recognize that policies and organizational adjustments play a significant role in reducing linguistic and administrative barriers in healthcare. These efforts are just as important as enhancing the cultural competency of healthcare professionals. To achieve cultural competence throughout the organization, it is crucial for policies to effectively address the concerns of individuals at all levels, ranging from senior management to clinicians, office workers, and administrative personnel (Chiu, 2009).

6.8. Health Communication Campaigns

A communication campaign is defined as the deliberate effort to achieve specific outcomes or effects in a significant number of individuals within a specified timeframe, using a structured series of communication activities. Communication campaigns can be differentiated from educational interventions that are specifically targeted towards individuals, whether it be in their own homes or through clinical or other established institutions (Snyder, 2007). We focus on a specific subset of campaigns that have large target populations, such as the entire population of a state or nation. However, it is important to note that the programs in this category exhibit significant variations. Here are a few common traits that are often observed, although they may not be universally present:

- The goal of communication campaigns is to directly educate individuals who are anticipated to adopt or transition to more favorable behaviors.
- Campaigns have the objective of making a substantial impact on a wide range of individuals, involving substantial resources such as

financial investments, volunteer efforts, and occasional collaborations with other organizations.

- Campaigns often utilize a range of media, combining personal media such as health professionals and outreach workers with mediated media like radio and television.
- The adoption of recommended behaviors is influenced by campaigns that aim to modify consumers' knowledge and beliefs about the behavior, as well as to change real and perceived social norms.
- Campaigns seek to enhance actual skills and self-confidence in performing the behavior (self-efficacy), as all of these factors are believed to impact behavior.
- Governments often provide financial support for campaigns, sometimes collaborating with private advocacy or professional associations.
- Campaigns often operate as components of broader social marketing initiatives. Social marketing involves the utilization of commercial marketing principles to tackle social and health concerns. Social marketing programs enhance communication efforts by incorporating additional elements of intervention (Snyder, 2007). A social marketing campaign focused on promoting childhood vaccination could assist a public communication campaign by implementing strategies such as offering vaccines at a discounted price, facilitating access to vaccines, or modifying the selection of vaccines that can be given together.
- In a broader sense, many campaigns aim to directly influence the population by also striving to modify public policy (such as taxes and regulations), other aspects of the environment and the economy, and the conduct of other social institutions. It can be inferred that these collaborative endeavors would have an indirect impact on populations. These multi-tiered social change initiatives may encompass activities such as developing and introducing new products, engaging in political and media advocacy, forming partnerships with private organizations, and mobilizing grassroots support. They comprehend the importance of the contextual and systemic constraints that either enable or hinder the desired modifications in behavior.

Communication campaigns have utilized a wide range of innovative methods to present compelling visuals that are credible, attractive, and appropriate for the intended audiences. Creating a distinctive and carefully crafted "signature" image or symbol, commonly known as "product branding" on social media, requires extensive research by numerous campaigns. This research aims to ensure that the picture or symbol effectively communicates and aligns with the cultural values of the intended audience. Although these campaigns are not very common, they have been successful in presenting stylish images that effectively resonate with their intended audiences (Snyder, 2007). In order to achieve this, they should capture the spotlight through their cutting-edge products, interactive technologies, influential figures, state-of-the-art innovations, and at times, thought-provoking advertisements.

6.9. The Importance of Ethical Considerations in Health Communication

The foundation of ethical healthcare lies in the practice of honest, courteous, clear, and compassionate communication. Ethics forms the fundamental basis of health communication. Various health communication initiatives, aimed at altering individuals' attitudes or behaviors regarding their health, encompass ethical considerations. Some examples of these actions include educating individuals about specific health concerns, promoting the adoption of healthy lifestyles, and serving as a role model of good behavior (Strasser & Gallagher, 1994). Health communication initiatives inevitably generate numerous ethical concerns, particularly when they address deeply ingrained social values and personal preferences, or when they aim to promote social norms that are opposed by specific groups.

The following are some ethical issues in health communication:

6.9.1. Informed Consent

In healthcare, there is a general consensus that obtaining informed consent from patients or their legal guardians is essential. In fact, in many healthcare systems, it is a legal obligation. However, this principle does not always apply to health communication. There is a lack of official guidelines for practitioners and scholars on how to obtain informed consent from communities for whom health messages are intended. Identifying an appropriate individual to serve as a representative for a specific population can be exceedingly challenging, particularly when dealing with a large group or community (Strasser & Gallagher, 1994). Moreover, within a group, certain individuals may perceive the health messages as objectionable, whereas others may desire their widespread dissemination. Utilizing advisory boards is a strategy commonly employed by governments or funding organizations to obtain informed consent in community or population settings. This technique presents an ethical quandary concerning the possibility of board members either not adequately representing marginalized groups or hindering the effectiveness of the communication intervention.

6.9.2. The Use of Persuasive Appeals

Health communication experts have developed theoretical and strategic methods for crafting persuasive statements and appeals that successfully influence individuals to adopt health-promoting beliefs and behaviors. Given that a persuasive method is inherently an effort to convince someone, it has the potential to infringe upon that individual's entitlement to be exempt from manipulation. Therefore, ethical considerations are deeply embedded in every strategy (Strasser & Gallagher, 1994). Many health communicators believe that using highly persuasive strategies is the most efficient method to encourage individuals to adhere to recommended health practices.

6.9.3. Communications Regarding Personal Responsibility

Personal responsibility is a concept that can be viewed as a representation of individuals' independence, but it also raises ethical quandaries that can be characterized as acts of victimization. The concept of responsibility encompasses obligations such as ensuring the well-being of one's spouse by promoting a healthy lifestyle and engaging in conversations about drugs with one's children. These messages fulfill moral responsibilities towards others and may be linked to social obligations. Being responsible entails making prudent choices regarding one's dietary habits, utilization of leisure time, and interpersonal interactions.

Individuals may be cautioned that leading irresponsible lifestyles could result in them becoming a liability to their families or society as a whole. An important ethical concern arises from the potential of these appeals to induce feelings of guilt and shame among individuals who are unable to adhere to the guidelines due to various reasons. Victim blaming refers to the situation where an individual's health choices are often influenced by external factors (e.g., pollution, employment and housing conditions, healthcare accessibility) rather than their own volition (Strasser & Gallagher, 1994). Therefore, messages of responsibility generate concerns regarding violations of the principle of "not causing harm". In addition, this sentiment can exert influence on public opinion and health policy, resulting in individuals who are deemed "irresponsible" being subjected to higher costs for certain medical conditions or receiving lower priority in accessing healthcare.

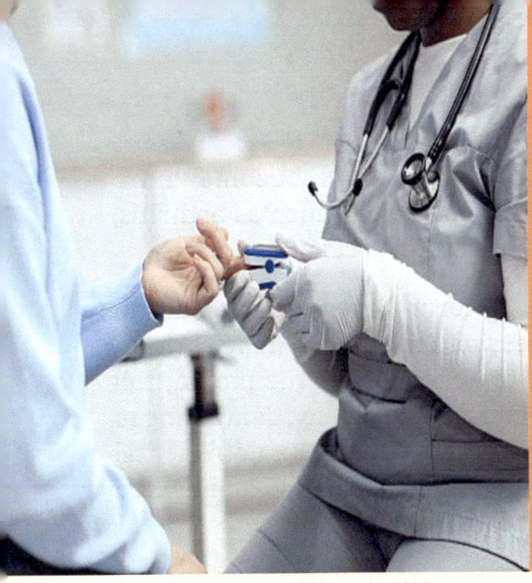

Chapter 7

HEALTH PROMOTION AND CHRONIC DISEASE PREVENTION

Contents

Chronic diseases or ailments are characterized by their prolonged duration, often lasting for an extended period of time. These illnesses often result in prolonged consequences that extend beyond a duration of three months. Common chronic diseases include diabetes, rheumatoid arthritis, asthma, chronic obstructive pulmonary disease (COPD), and autoimmune illnesses. Various bodily parts can be affected and go through periods of improvement and recurrence. Chronic diseases have a significant impact on global mortality, accounting for more than 63% of all fatalities.

7.1. The Impact of Chronic Diseases

Chronic diseases such as diabetes, heart disease, stroke, and cancer continue to be significant contributors to morbidity and mortality on a global scale. Throughout the early 1900s, there was a notable transition from infectious diseases to noncommunicable diseases, which has persisted to this day. In recent times, with the increase in life expectancy, there has been a rise in the prevalence and cost of chronic diseases. According to a study conducted by Mascie-Taylor and Karim in 2003, it is estimated that by 2030, chronic illness will have a significant impact on the global economy, with a projected cost of $47 trillion. Community-based and individual lifestyle choices and behaviors play a crucial role in the development and management of chronic illnesses. Several diseases, such as diabetes, heart disease, and respiratory disorders, are strongly influenced by certain risk factors. These risk factors include lack of physical activity, unhealthy eating habits, smoking, and excessive alcohol intake. Unfortunately, when considering lifestyle and socioeconomic determinants of health, prevention continues to receive less funding compared to treatment. In order to effectively address the projected trajectory of chronic illness, it is imperative that we focus on innovation in drugs and technology, while also making a significant investment in prevention. This is a crucial factor that will shape our future.

Chronic illnesses affect millions of individuals around the globe, placing a significant strain on healthcare systems.

7.1.1. Impacts That Chronic Illnesses Have on Individuals

Physical limitations can greatly impact one's mobility, freedom, and overall quality of life. These limitations are often a result of the physical disabilities that chronic diseases can bring about. Everyday tasks become more challenging due to conditions such as arthritis, chronic pain, and cardiovascular disorders.

Managing a long-term illness can result in feelings of depression, anxiety, and hopelessness. It is important to acknowledge the mental toll that comes with this responsibility. Continuing to grapple with symptoms can have a detrimental effect on one's mental well-being, as highlighted by Mascie-Taylor and Karim (2003).

People who have long-term illnesses often find themselves avoiding social situations due to feelings of discomfort, exhaustion, or the fear of being stigmatized. Experiencing solitude exacerbates the burden of their emotions.

7.1.2. Chronic Illnesses and Economic Impacts

The cost of healthcare can be significantly impacted by chronic disorders. Public health and private health budgets face significant strain due to the high number of medical visits, prescription drugs, and specialty therapies. Chronic illnesses can have a significant impact on both employees and employers, leading to absenteeism and decreased productivity at work (Mascie-Taylor & Karim, 2003). There are additional financial implications that extend beyond the expenses associated with healthcare. Taking care of a family member or friend with a chronic illness can be challenging, as it involves dealing with emotional, physical, and financial strain.

7.1.3. Chronic Illnesses and Societal Burden

The prevalence of chronic illnesses puts a strain on healthcare systems, diverting funds from acute care and preventative measures. Managing chronic illnesses poses a significant challenge for clinics, hospitals, and primary care institutions (Mascie-Taylor & Karim, 2003). One important aspect to consider is the impact on the workforce. Individuals who are afflicted with chronic illnesses tend to exhibit decreased productivity, elevated rates of absenteeism, and an inclination to retire earlier than their healthier counterparts. Ensuring the productivity and well-being of employees poses a significant challenge for employers.

Acute outbreaks and emergencies compete for attention alongside chronic diseases. Allocating funds towards management and prevention necessitates a delicate equilibrium.

7.1.4. Preventive Strategies for Chronic Illnesses

Health Education: Health education plays a crucial role in disseminating information about lifestyle changes, early identification, and risk factors. The initial step towards prevention involves making informed decisions. Policy Interventions: Policy interventions play a crucial role in addressing chronic diseases. Governments can prioritize prevention by enacting laws that promote wholesome settings, ensure easy access to nutritious food, and encourage physical exercise (Mascie-Taylor & Karim, 2003). Research and Innovation: Research and innovation play a crucial role in improving healthcare. Personalized care, the development of novel treatments, and conducting research on chronic illnesses are all important areas that can help alleviate the burden of healthcare.

7.2. Factors That Contribute to the Development of Chronic Diseases

In order to effectively manage and reduce these disorders, it is crucial to recognize and tackle the risk factors that play a role in their development. Below is a list of ten common risk factors associated with chronic illnesses:

7.2.1. Physical Inactivity

Physical inactivity has been associated with an elevated risk of obesity, type 2 diabetes, and cardiovascular diseases. Regular physical activity has been shown to have numerous benefits for our overall health. It can enhance blood sugar control, aid in weight management, and promote cardiovascular well-being. By engaging in regular physical activity, we can reduce the risk of developing these health issues.

People who lead sedentary lifestyles are at a higher risk of developing chronic illnesses that are associated with lack of physical activity (Steyn & Damasceno, 2006). Factors such as the presence of secure recreational spaces, affordable fitness centers, and community programs play a significant role in influencing an individual's ability to engage in regular exercise.

7.2.2. Excessive Alcohol Consumption

Excessive alcohol consumption significantly increases the likelihood of developing heart problems, liver diseases, and certain forms of cancer. Heavy drinkers make up the majority of individuals who are at risk for developing chronic alcohol-related disorders.

The social determinants that influence drinking patterns include cultural perspectives on alcohol consumption, the availability of alcohol based on local regulations and accessibility, and economic factors such as employment status and financial stability that can affect drinking habits and purchasing power (Steyn & Damasceno, 2006). When considering effective interventions, it is crucial to take into account the cultural and economic factors alongside providing information and support for responsible alcohol consumption.

7.2.3. Tobacco Use

Tobacco use greatly increases the risk of developing chronic illnesses such as heart disease, chronic obstructive pulmonary disease (COPD), and lung cancer. Tobacco smoke contains substances that have been found to have negative effects on the body. These effects include inflammation, narrowing of blood vessels, and damage to lung tissue (Steyn & Damasceno, 2006). People who engage in heavy smoking or are frequently exposed to secondhand smoke have a higher risk of developing chronic illnesses.

7.2.4. Unhealthy Diet

Consuming excessive amounts of processed foods, sugary beverages, and saturated fats is associated with an unhealthy diet. This can lead to a higher likelihood of developing obesity, type 2 diabetes, heart disease, and various forms of cancer. Chronic diseases related to diet are often found in individuals who have unhealthy eating habits. These habits are often influenced by factors like low income, limited access to nutritious foods in their communities, and food insecurity (Steyn & Damasceno, 2006). Addressing socioeconomic variables involves various strategies such as enhancing food security, increasing access to nutritious foods, and offering nutrition education in disadvantaged areas.

7.2.5. Air Pollution

Air pollution, particularly fine particulate matter and toxic pollutants, has been linked to respiratory diseases like asthma and COPD, heart diseases, and certain types of cancer. Populations residing in regions with elevated levels of air pollution, impacted by urbanization and industrial activity, face a heightened vulnerability to chronic diseases associated with pollution (Steyn & Damasceno, 2006). Other factors that are closely linked to social determinants are the geographical location of housing, disparities in economic conditions, and the policies related to the environment.

7.2.6. Inherited Mutations

Inherited mutations can increase the likelihood of developing various genetic diseases and disorders. As an example, it is worth noting that mutations in the CFTR gene can lead to the development of cystic fibrosis. Similarly, mutations in the BRCA1 and BRCA2 genes have been associated with an elevated risk of breast and ovarian cancer. Early cancer detection and genetic testing play a crucial role in halting the progression of numerous chronic conditions.

7.2.7. Family History

Individuals with a family history of chronic illnesses are at a higher risk, often due to the transmission of genetic and environmental factors within families. Family history can contribute to an elevated risk of various diseases, including heart disease, stroke, certain types of cancer (such as breast, lung, and colon cancer), and genetic disorders. It is important to note that taking preventive measures, such as regular checkups, early screenings, and adopting a healthy lifestyle, can play a significant role in reducing the impact of these predispositions (Steyn & Damasceno, 2006). Early detection and prevention are greatly influenced by various social factors, including health education and the availability of healthcare services. It is crucial for individuals with a family history of chronic illness to prioritize routine tests and education in healthcare practices.

7.2.8. The Rural Location

Living in a remote area can result in limited access to medical care facilities and resources, potentially causing delays in the diagnosis and treatment of chronic illnesses. Improving access to healthcare can be achieved by implementing transportation services and establishing Rural

Health Clinics (RHCs). Additionally, educating individuals about risk factors in rural communities is crucial for enhancing healthcare access (Steyn & Damasceno, 2006).

7.2.9. Gender

Gender can play a significant role in determining the likelihood of developing a chronic illness, as certain diseases may impact men and women in distinct ways. It is worth noting that there is a higher prevalence of heart disease among men, while women tend to be more vulnerable to conditions such as ovarian and breast cancer (Steyn & Damasceno, 2006). Understanding the risks associated with a specific gender and following recommended screening protocols and lifestyle changes are proactive measures.

7.2.10. Low Socioeconomic Status

There is a strong correlation between low socioeconomic level and various negative health outcomes. Factors such as inadequate nutrition, heightened stress levels, and limited healthcare access contribute to an increased risk of developing chronic illnesses including diabetes, heart disease, and mental health issues (Steyn & Damasceno, 2006). Prevention methods encompass a range of initiatives aimed at addressing economic inequities, providing social assistance, and improving access to healthcare services.

7.3. Lifestyle Interventions for Chronic Disease Prevention

There are some dietary and lifestyle changes that have been shown to decrease the likelihood of developing chronic diseases.

7.3.1. Avoid Tobacco Use

Preventing the initiation of smoking or encouraging cessation for those who already smoke is of utmost importance in the prevention of CVD and cancer (Gaziano et al., 2007). By refraining from using smokeless tobacco, you can significantly reduce your risk of developing oral cancer.

7.3.2. Maintain a Healthy Weight

On a global scale, there has been a rapid increase in the prevalence of obesity. Overweight, with a body mass index (BMI) of 25 to 30, is actually more prevalent and carries greater risks of various diseases, despite receiving less attention compared to obesity, which is defined as a BMI of 30 or above. As an illustration, individuals who are overweight (with a BMI greater than 23) face a significantly higher risk of developing coronary artery disease (CAD) and hypertension, with the risk being two to three times greater compared to those who have a lean body. Additionally, the risk of developing type 2 diabetes is more than ten times higher for overweight individuals (Gaziano et al., 2007). Higher death rates are observed in both overweight and obese individuals for colon, breast (postmenopausal), renal, endometrial, and other malignancies.

Even though they may not be classified as overweight, a considerable number of individuals with a BMI below 25 have experienced substantial weight gain since their early adulthood. As a result, they are also more prone to these illnesses. As an example, it is worth noting that the occurrence of hypertension was significantly higher among individuals with a BMI of around 25 compared to the leanest individuals in rural China. In this particular region, both men and women had an average BMI of less than 21 (Gaziano et al., 2007). In recent times, there has been a broadening of the definition of overweight in Asia. This expansion now includes individuals with a BMI of 23 to 25. The reason behind this change is the growing number of Asians who are experiencing the detrimental consequences of carrying excess body fat, even with a BMI below 25.

Waist circumference serves as a valuable metric for assessing the accumulation of abdominal fat and offers supplementary insights. Multiple studies have consistently shown that waist circumference remains a strong predictor of CAD, stroke, and type 2 diabetes, even when accounting for BMI. According to current guidelines, in the United States, it is considered healthy for males to have a waist circumference of approximately 100 centimeters, while women should aim for around 88 centimeters. Nevertheless, for numerous individuals, the amount of abdominal fat mentioned would exceed what is considered ideal, as stated by Gaziano, et al., in 2007. Given the simplicity of measuring belly circumference, even in situations where scales are not available, it would be advantageous to conduct further research in order to establish standards that are relevant to specific regions.

It is worth considering that factors beyond the macronutrient composition of food may be contributing to the global obesity crisis. Across many nations, there has been a significant increase in the availability of inexpensive food energy obtained from sugar, vegetable oils, and processed cereals. Food producers and suppliers utilize carefully planned methods to craft products that are both convenient and visually appealing, all while using affordable ingredients.

7.3.3. Maintain Daily Physical Activity

In modern wealthy nations, people's opportunities to exert energy have significantly decreased. This is evident in various aspects of their lives, such as commuting, work, and even at home. Developing nations are also witnessing significant decreases in physical activity as a result of urbanization, the increasing availability of motorized transportation that is replacing walking and cycling, and the automation of work. However, it is crucial to emphasize that maintaining a healthy weight and preventing obesity are strongly influenced by engaging in regular physical activity (Gaziano et al., 2007). As an example, it has been observed that increasing physical activity, such as walking, is associated with a decrease in BMI among middle-aged West African women. Similarly, in China, individuals who own cars have a significantly higher risk of obesity, with an 80% increase compared to those who do not own cars.

Regular physical activity has been shown to have numerous health benefits. It can help reduce the risk of conditions such as CAD, stroke, type 2 diabetes, colon and breast cancer, osteoporotic fractures, osteoarthritis, depression, and erectile dysfunction. Additionally, it plays a crucial role in maintaining a healthy weight (Gaziano et al., 2007). Engaging in a mere 30 minutes of daily walking has been found to have noteworthy health advantages. Nevertheless, engaging in longer and more rigorous physical activity is associated with even greater reductions in risk.

Research has shown a clear connection between the daily duration of television viewing and increased rates of obesity in both adults and children. Additionally, individuals who spend excessive time in front of the TV are at a greater risk of developing gallstones and type 2 diabetes. One possible explanation for this correlation could be a decrease in physical activity and an increase in the consumption of high-calorie foods and beverages, which are often heavily advertised on television. It has been found that decreasing the amount of time spent watching television can result in weight loss. In fact, the American Academy of Pediatrics recommends that individuals should not exceed two hours of television viewing per day.

7.3.4. Eat a Healthy Diet

- **Substitute Saturated and Trans Fats with Unsaturated Fats, Which Include Sources of Omega-3 Fatty Acids:** One way to reduce the risk of CAD is by replacing saturated fats with unsaturated fats, which can help lower LDL cholesterol levels in the blood. In addition, it is worth noting that polyunsaturated fats have the potential to lower the risk of severe coronary artery disease by effectively preventing ventricular arrhythmias. The fats mentioned here are the long-chain omega-3 fish oils and alpha-linoleic acid, which is the main omega-3 fatty acid found in plants (Gaziano et al., 2007). In a case-control study conducted in Costa Rica, it was found that individuals who had a high intake of alpha-linoleic acid experienced a significant 80% decrease in the risk of myocardial infarction. This finding is particularly interesting considering the low consumption of fish in Costa Rica. It is worth noting that in several cultures, the consumption of omega 3 fatty acids is often insufficient, particularly among those who have limited intake of seafood and rely on low-quality primary oils such as partly hydrogenated soybean, corn, sunflower, or palm oil.
- **Ensure Generous Consumption of Fruits and Vegetables and Adequate Folic Acid Intake:** Consuming a substantial amount of fruit and vegetables has been extensively correlated with a reduced risk of stroke and CAD. Part of this effect can be attributed to higher potassium intakes, with folic acid also likely playing a role. Supplementing with folic acid has been shown to reduce the risk of neural tube defects during pregnancy (Gaziano et al., 2007). Furthermore, a significant amount of research suggests that the consumption of multiple vitamins containing folic acid can reduce the likelihood of developing colon and potentially breast cancer. Conversely, a diet low in folic acid has been associated with a higher risk of these types of cancers. The findings connecting folic acid intake to cardiovascular disease and certain types of cancer have important implications for many developing countries. There is a significant lack of fruit and vegetable consumption in numerous regions. As an example, it is worth noting that a significant portion of the adult population in northern China has a deficiency in Folic acid.
- **Consume Cereal Products in Their Whole-Grain, High-Fiber Form:** There are a couple of benefits to incorporating whole, high-fiber cereals into your diet. Consuming fiber from cereal products has consistently been associated with a reduced risk of type 2 diabetes and CAD. One possible explanation for this association is the natural properties of fiber found in whole grains, along with the presence of vitamins and minerals. Consuming excessive amounts of refined carbohydrates significantly increases the risk of developing type 2 diabetes and CAD, while also

worsening the metabolic syndrome (Gaziano et al., 2007). Additionally, increasing your intake of dietary fiber has been found to be beneficial in preventing constipation and managing weight.

- **Limit Consumption of Sugar and Sugar-Based Beverages:** Sugar provides no significant nutritional benefits aside from its calorie content. It is derived from sources such as sugarcane, sugar beets, or high-fructose corn syrups. Therefore, it presents a significant health issue for individuals who are already susceptible to obesity. In addition, it is important to note that the consumption of sugar can significantly increase the glycemic load of one's diet. This, in turn, can worsen metabolic syndrome and significantly elevate the risk of developing diabetes and CAD (Gaziano et al., 2007). It is important to note that the World Health Organization (WHO) has advised limiting sugar intake to a maximum of 10% of energy. However, it is generally recommended to consume even less sugar due to the potential negative effects on metabolism and the fact that it provides empty calories.
- **Limit Excessive Caloric Intake from Any Source:** It is crucial to prioritize conserving energy from all sources, particularly when considering the significant impact that obesity and overweight have on the development of numerous chronic diseases (Gaziano et al., 2007). It is of utmost importance to decrease the consumption of sugar-sweetened beverages due to the fact that the calories in drinks are not as closely regulated as those in solid food.
- **It is Important to Restrict the Consumption of Sodium:** The justification for limiting sodium intake primarily stems from its effect on blood pressure, a major risk factor for coronary heart disease and stroke (Gaziano et al., 2007). The World Health Organization has recommended a daily maximum of 1.7 grams of sodium (or 5 grams of salt).

7.4. Screening and Early Detection of Chronic Diseases

In cases where individuals do not display any noticeable symptoms, a screening test is conducted to detect potential illnesses or health concerns. The primary objective is to minimize the likelihood of illness or detect it at an early stage to ensure optimal treatment through timely identification, adjustments in lifestyle, or vigilant monitoring (Fragala et al., 2019). Screening tests are utilized to identify a specific group of individuals who may require additional testing to determine the presence or absence of a disease. However, it is important to note that these tests are not considered diagnostic tools.

Below are some of the common screening tests:

7.4.1. Cholesterol Measurements

One of the methods employed in medical practice is blood testing, which serves the purpose of screening for cholesterol levels. Having blood cholesterol readings that exceed the normal range can significantly elevate the chances of developing CVD. Studies have shown that individuals with high cholesterol can reduce their risk of heart disease by lowering their cholesterol levels (Fragala et al., 2019). It is important to understand that having cholesterol levels within the normal range does not necessarily mean that heart disease is absent.

7.4.2. Fecal Occult Blood Test

Chemical testing or microscopic examination can be used to identify fecal occult blood, which is the presence of hemoglobin in the stool. When blood is found in the stool, it could indicate the presence of a malignant growth associated with colorectal cancer. For the test, it is necessary to collect three stool samples and carefully examine them under a microscope to check for the presence of blood (Fragala et al., 2019). It is important to understand that there are various non-cancerous factors that can lead to the presence of blood in a stool sample. These factors include certain foods or medications, gastrointestinal bleeding, or hemorrhoids.

7.4.3. Pap Test (Also Called Pap Smears)

Cell samples are collected from the cervixes of women for Pap screenings. These screenings are conducted to detect any cellular abnormalities that may be indicative of cervical cancer.

The Pap smear is an essential screening tool for sexually active women under 65. It plays a crucial role in identifying cancer at an early stage, even when symptoms are not present (Fragala et al., 2019). It is important to understand that a "abnormal" Pap smear does not necessarily mean that an individual has cervical cancer. Furthermore, it is recommended by various organizations to conduct HPV (human papilloma virus) screening in certain populations during Pap smears.

7.4.4. Prostate Specific Antigen (PSA)

This blood test is used to determine the levels of prostate specific antigen (PSA) in the blood. Antigens are substances that trigger a response from the immune system. Prostate cancer can lead to elevated levels of the prostate-specific antigen. It is important to understand that there are certain prostate disorders, such as benign prostatic hyperplasia (BPH), which is a noncancerous enlargement of the prostate, that can also lead to an elevation in PSA levels (Fragala et al., 2019).

7.4.5. Mammography

It is recommended by various organizations, such as the USPSTF, that women over the age of 50 undergo mammography screening for breast cancer on a yearly to biennial basis. This examination is performed in conjunction with a clinical breast exam.

7.4.6. Diabetes or Prediabetes

It is important to note that screening for diabetes or prediabetes should commence for all adults at the age of 45, regardless of their weight (Fragala et al., 2019). Furthermore, individuals who are overweight or obese and possess one or more additional risk factors for diabetes should undergo examination, even in the absence of any noticeable symptoms of the disease.

7.5. Managing Chronic Diseases

People with a chronic illness may need to actively manage their condition for the rest of their lives. It is within the power of every individual to proactively take charge of their own health. Treatment for the symptoms of a chronic illness can potentially enhance one's quality of life.

To effectively manage a chronic condition, it is important to maintain a healthy lifestyle which involves proper nutrition, regular exercise, and sufficient sleep. Additionally, it is crucial to follow the prescribed medication regimen and adhere to any management plans provided (Landon et al., 2007). Finally, it is important to schedule regular meetings with your general practitioner or specialist.

Medicare provides funding for the implementation of plans aimed at managing chronic diseases. These programs provide assistance to individuals in need of ongoing treatment from a team of medical experts, along with a structured approach to managing a long-term health condition.

Properly managing your chronic illness can have numerous benefits:

By focusing on improving your overall health and well-being, you can proactively prevent or delay potential challenges and slow down the progression of your illness.

There are several healthcare providers who may be involved in your treatment include specialists and allied health professionals. These could include the following examples.

- A social worker provides guidance and information on various public and private assistance programs.
- A dietitian provides professional guidance on food and nutrition.
- An occupational therapist help you maintain, regain, or improve your independence.
- If you are currently experiencing any discomfort or difficulty with your mobility, it would be advisable to seek the assistance of a qualified physiotherapist. They possess the expertise to address and alleviate such concerns.
- Consulting a psychologist can be beneficial in managing the challenges that come with a chronic disease.

It is important to note that adopting a healthy lifestyle can greatly assist in effectively managing a chronic illness. One of the key elements of leading a healthy lifestyle is to ensure that you maintain a healthy weight. It is also important to refrain from smoking and engage in regular physical activity to the best of your ability. Additionally, getting enough sleep and limiting alcohol consumption are crucial factors in promoting overall well-being (Landon et al., 2007). It is important to acknowledge and understand the impact that medications can have on our bodies. By following the prescribed instructions, we can ensure that we are taking them in the most effective and appropriate manner. It is important for individuals to regularly consult with their doctor to ensure that the medications they are taking for long periods of time are still suitable (Landon et al., 2007).

7.6. Role of Healthcare Providers in Chronic Disease Prevention

Healthcare providers play a crucial role in preventing chronic diseases. They have the knowledge and expertise to make a significant impact on the health of individuals. By implementing preventive measures, healthcare providers can help reduce the burden of chronic diseases and improve overall well-being.

7.6.1. Enhancing Accessibility

In order to enhance accessibility to care, it would be beneficial to introduce schedule adjustments, after-hours care, and/or avenues for consultation. Providers develop and implement strategies to improve access to care, adjusting them based on patient needs and preferences (Hawk et al., 2012). One effective way to enhance accessibility is by offering after-hours and same-day appointments. Additionally, providing phone consultations with certified health experts and allowing consultations by email, text, or other technology can also be beneficial.

7.6.2. Care Management

Effective management and coordination of patient care in complex and challenging situations. Practices are responsible for identifying patients who may pose a risk, developing team-based treatment plans to ensure they receive the appropriate care, coordinating any necessary outside resources, and closely monitoring the progress of patients. Providers modify their responses according to the health hazards identified by their patients.

7.6.3. Team-Based Care Coordination

The practices identify a multidisciplinary care team consisting of doctors, nurses, medical assistants, pharmacists, social workers, and other clinical professionals. Practices incorporate specific strategies to facilitate collaboration within their operational model. This can include scheduling case conferences, coordinating activities, and promoting communication among the team members responsible for a patient's care (Hawk et al., 2012). In addition, practices establish mechanisms to coordinate with external entities such as hospitals, urgent care facilities, outpatient specialists, community services, rehabilitation facilities, and the patient's support network. Coordination plays a crucial role in enhancing care planning, diagnosis, treatment, management during care transitions, and patient coaching to improve treatment adherence. This capability allows for the integration of behavioral health and primary care practices.

7.6.4. Patient Engagement

Medication management, health coaching, and outreach are important aspects to consider in healthcare. Health care providers strive to develop a culture that is dedicated to understanding and addressing patient needs. In addition, they offer a comprehensive self-management curriculum and a range of tools to promote patient engagement. One possible approach is to educate patients, provide incentives, and utilize technology (Hawk et al., 2012). Practices develop and implement patient engagement programs with a particular emphasis on high-risk patients.

7.6.5. Health IT Enablement

Healthcare providers utilize various health IT resources, including practice management software, electronic health records, and data from DHIN, to effectively coordinate care. This enables them to maximize the availability and connectivity of clinical and claims data, facilitating coordinated care (Hawk et al., 2012). Practices enhance the growth of the Community Health Record by incorporating clinical data, integrating health IT into their workflow, and effectively analyzing data.

7.7. Policy Initiatives for Chronic Disease Prevention

Enhancing well-being operates based on six policy statements. This aims to enhance health by fostering collaboration among employers, government agencies, community organizations, individuals, and healthcare professionals. It is a comprehensive, long-term approach that requires the collective effort of all stakeholders.

7.7.1. The First Policy Statement

This involves self-management. It focuses on assuming responsibility for one's own well-being. Individuals who actively engage in the daily management of their diseases often experience enhanced health and an elevated quality of life (Bunnell et al., 2012). Taking care of one's health is crucial in reducing the transmission of illnesses, preventing complications, and potentially reducing the need for hospitalization.

Individuals living with chronic illnesses can be empowered to play a more active role in managing their health through the provision of suitable educational resources and support from both their community and healthcare providers. Gaining new knowledge, skills, and confidence enables individuals to effectively manage their symptoms and lead a more wholesome lifestyle (Bunnell et al., 2012). The patient has the ultimate authority to decide when and if they want to become more involved in their healthcare. By working alongside a healthcare professional, they can acquire the information and confidence needed to take charge of their own health.

There are various ways to provide support for self-management, including web-based modules, video conferencing, telemedicine, government and community-based group programs, and self-help materials. Through the application of these techniques, individuals acquire the skills to effectively address challenges, set personal health goals, analyze relevant information to make well-informed decisions regarding their well-being, engage in meaningful conversations with healthcare providers, and successfully implement changes to improve their overall health.

7.7.2. The Second Policy Statement

This policy statement is a focus on prevention and awareness. Promoting health through widespread initiatives is crucial in the prevention of disease. Collaboration among individuals, communities, and the medical system is crucial for the advancement of wellness and health (Bunnell et al., 2012). To foster the well-being of individuals and communities, partners have the opportunity to enhance neighborhood initiatives, develop health-conscious public policies, and create conducive environments. The main objectives of initiatives that focus on these aspects are to:

- Increase physical activity
- Promote a healthy diet
- Reduce risk factors for chronic diseases

7.7.3. The Third Policy Statement

Health care delivery involves the organization and coordination of services to effectively meet the needs of individuals.

Chronic illnesses encompass a wide range of conditions that are complex and have multiple aspects to consider. It is imperative to implement reforms in the structure and provision of health care in order to ensure optimal treatment for individuals with chronic illnesses or those at risk of developing them. Expanding the area of practice as necessary and outlining the obligations and functions of healthcare professionals are essential components of this process.

Restructuring the delivery of care and implementing new practice models are essential for meeting the unique needs of each individual (Bunnell et al., 2012). In addition, it involves the coordination of healthcare professionals to efficiently connect individuals with the necessary resources in a timely manner.

For the effective prevention and management of chronic illness, it is crucial to have a long-term commitment and a well-organized strategy for care. Improving the quality of care can be accomplished through the implementation of a collaborative approach. A variety of healthcare professionals, such as nurses, pharmacists, social workers, home health aides, nutritionists, physiotherapists, doctors, and more, have the ability to come together and create collaborative teams. The composition of the healthcare team can be adjusted and customized to meet the unique needs of every patient, as discussed by Bunnell, et al. (2012). The medical team works together with the patient and their family to accomplish specific health goals. In this approach, the focus is on making illness prevention and health promotion standard procedures.

7.7.4. The Fourth Policy Statement

The fourth policy statement focuses on practice guidelines. Utilizing up-to-date information and adhering to established standards in order to deliver high-quality care. For the successful prevention and treatment of chronic illness, it is essential to apply a recommended set of principles. Health care providers have access to up-to-date advice on the diagnosis, treatment, management, and prevention of specific diseases through practice guidelines. The recommendations are based on best practices in client care and are supported by recent research. Establishing and implementing practice guidelines is essential to ensuring consistency in healthcare and decision-making throughout the province. When developing provincial guidelines, it is important to carefully consider both the clinical and financial effectiveness. The decisions made must be informed by the data that is available. Healthcare providers, health-based groups, and health research agencies play a crucial role in the development and approval of provincial practice guidelines (Bunnell et al., 2012).

7.7.5. The Fifth Policy Statement

This is a focus on information systems and research. The process of gathering and analyzing data to effectively guide and monitor programs and services.

Gathering data on the management and prevention of chronic illness can be done through various methods such as research, personal record audits, program and service assessments, and interviews with patients, families, and caregivers (Bunnell et al., 2012). A deeper comprehension of chronic diseases allows healthcare professionals and legislators to create more effective policies, programs, and services, ultimately enhancing their ability to provide optimal care for individuals.

7.7.6. The Sixth Policy Statement

The sixth policy statement focuses on community action. Collaborating for improved health outcomes.

The level of support provided by a person's community has a significant impact on their ability to maintain good health.

The community is comprised of various entities such as the municipal and provincial governments, neighborhood associations, businesses, medical facilities, educational institutions, places of worship, and all citizens. Communities have the ability to provide support to individuals and families in order to help them lead healthy lives. This can be achieved through the implementation of various policies, initiatives, and services (Bunnell et al., 2012).

Examples of initiatives that can be implemented include the creation of smoke-free areas, promotion of local food production, opportunities for skill- and knowledge-sharing, establishment of safe spaces for physical activity, and setting a positive example of healthy living in various settings.

7.8. Community-Based Chronic Disease Prevention Programs

Community support affects health. The community includes municipal and provincial governments, neighborhood associations, businesses, medical facilities, educational institutions, places of worship, and citizens. Communities can help families live healthy lives through policies, initiatives, and services. Creating smoke-free areas, encouraging local food production, providing opportunities for skill- and knowledge-sharing, providing safe spaces for physical activity, and demonstrating healthy living at work, in the open, and in open spaces are examples.

Steps to a HealthierUS (now Healthy Communities program) from the Centers for Disease Control and Prevention (CDC) funds communities to identify and improve environmental factors and policies that affect health to reduce obesity and other chronic diseases and encourage people to avoid tobacco, eat healthy, and exercise. This and other publicly-funded programs have supported successful community-based interventions including those listed below.

The Steps program in the Alabama River Region trained diabetes wellness advocates to help individuals manage their disease and set health goals. Patients who visited the ER less than half as often between 2004 and 2007.

To overcome barriers to breast and cervical cancer screenings for African American women over 40, the Alabama REACH 2010 Breast and Cervical Cancer Coalition (ABCCC) created a community action plan. The strategy included a core working group of volunteers and medical experts and grants to nonprofit organizations that provided screenings, outreach, and educational materials. The intervention increased mammogram use by 14% in the two years after its implementation. Moreover, 11% more women had Pap tests within two years of the intervention. Eight counties introduced a patient navigation system to reduce the mammography screening gap between black and white patients.

Alaska has historically had higher rates of cigarette and chewing tobacco use than the rest of the country. To address this health issue, the Alaska Department of Health and Social Services created a comprehensive tobacco control program based on the CDC's Best Practices for Comprehensive Tobacco Control Programs—2007. The program includes counter marketing, community-based initiatives, youth and educational initiatives, secondhand smoke elimination, health disparities, quitting, a free quit line, and evaluation. Since 2002, thousands of Alaskans have called the quit line, and 40% had quit by 2007. Alaska has improved due to its efforts. The 2008 Alaska Behavioral Risk Factor Surveillance System showed a tobacco use decline. CCAA is an environmental and social justice movement in Arizona aimed at reducing high-risk drinking among college students (18–24 years old) and its negative effects. The action was developed at Northern Illinois University with Arizona University input. Among other methods, the CCAA runs a campus-wide media campaign to dispel alcohol myths and discourage drinking. Post-CCAA implementation (1995–1998), freshmen's weekly alcohol use dropped from 43% to 31% ($p < .01$), and those who had five or more drinks per occasion in the past two weeks decreased from 43% to 31%.

7.9. Integrating Mental Health in Chronic Disease Prevention

Optimal mental wellbeing, also known as mental health, mitigates the likelihood of health-compromising behaviors and improves the outlook for individuals with chronic illnesses. The subsequent section emphasizes the most recent research on the crucial significance of mental health in chronic illness among young individuals. This examines the specific correlations between emotional experiences during childhood and physical health in adulthood, the connections between obesity, diabetes, and asthma, and the unique interplay between mental health, risk-taking behavior, and chronic disease.

7.9.1. Obesity

It is crucial to understand the correlations between obesity and mental health, considering the alarming statistic that more than 31% of children and teenagers are currently overweight or obese. There exists a reciprocal relationship between the two phenomena: obesity has an impact on mental health, while mental health also has an impact on obesity. Research shows that individuals who are overweight have a 55% higher risk of developing depression over time. Similarly, those who experience sadness are 58% more likely to become obese.

Obesity often leads to significant social and emotional challenges for young individuals. Obesity in youth is a significant public health concern that unfortunately carries a heavy burden of negative stereotypes and peer rejection. As a result, students who are overweight are at a higher risk of facing challenges such as anxiety, behavior issues, bullying, and feelings of inferiority and worthlessness (Lando et al., 2006). It is not surprising that the risk of an adolescent suicide attempt is higher among those who are overweight.

7.9.2. Asthma

Adolescents who are diagnosed with anxiety or depression often experience a significant increase in the severity of their asthma symptoms. These symptoms may include difficulty breathing, chest tightness, coughing, persistent colds, and wheezing when they are sick.

The presence of this co-morbidity carries significant implications. As evidenced by a study, it was discovered that high school students with asthma exhibited a similar or even higher rate of substance use that poses a health risk compared to their peers without asthma. Additionally, these students also experienced significantly higher rates of depressed thinking. It is worth noting that there was a significant increase in the occurrence of depressive symptoms, suicide ideation, planning, attempts, and injuries among individuals with asthma (Lando et al., 2006). In addition, it is worth noting that a higher proportion of students experiencing depression engaged in the use of substances that are known to have negative effects on health, such as alcohol, cocaine, marijuana, and tobacco, compared to high school students who have asthma. It is crucial to recognize the significance of addressing childhood asthma as more than a mere chronic illness.

7.9.3. Diabetes

In the last three decades, there has been a significant rise in the prevalence of childhood and young diabetes, particularly among minority populations. Identifying diabetes in young individuals, regardless of whether it is type 1 or type 2, poses considerable challenges across various aspects of life.

There appears to be a correlation between depression and diabetes in adults, with individuals who have depression being at a higher risk of developing diabetes, and those with diabetes being more prone to experiencing depression. However, the exact nature of this relationship is not yet fully comprehended. It is worth noting that depression is a commonly observed co-morbid condition in children and adolescents with type 1 or type 2 diabetes. Research suggests that around 12–18% of individuals with diabetes experience clinically significant symptoms of depression (Lando et al., 2006).

7.10. Future Prospects in Chronic Disease Prevention

The expansion of industrialization has led to a significant increase in the incidence of chronic diseases such as diabetes mellitus, hypertension, dyslipidemia, and cardiovascular disease. According to projections, the global diabetic population is expected to reach 552 million by 2030, which is an increase from 366 million in 2011 (Howse et al., 2020). Diabetes causes approximately 4.6 million deaths annually, making it a substantial healthcare challenge. In order to ensure effective and top-notch medical care, it is crucial to improve medical services, which unquestionably leads to increased demand and expenses. Failure to modify the existing system will inevitably result in additional occurrences of chronic disease and its related complications. Change incurs a social and financial expense that needs to be recognized. The primary emphasis of contemporary healthcare systems is on treatment-oriented care. It is crucial to redirect attention towards the prevention of chronic diseases. Healthy individuals with a high risk of developing health problems need education on managing their lifestyle. This includes providing them with guidance on diet and exercise routines (Howse et al., 2020). Current medical systems are insufficient in terms of temporal, geographical, and financial resources to adequately address lifestyle factors. Every diabetic individual must integrate dietary and exercise regimens into their daily routines.

The introduction of these requirements prompted the creation of multiple U-healthcare systems and the assessment of their therapeutic advantages. The term "ubiquitous" refers to something that is present at all times and in all places. When this term is combined with "healthcare," it creates the commonly used term "ubiquitous healthcare," or "U-healthcare." U-healthcare ensures universal access to medical services or healthcare at any location and time, utilizing both mobile and fixed networking. The interest in u-healthcare is increasing due to the recognition that chronic illnesses require continuous treatment that is integrated into daily life (Howse et al., 2020). Treatment approaches that focus primarily on hospitals are ineffective in managing such disorders.

Efficiently reducing healthcare expenses while maintaining high standards is of utmost importance. Diabetes patients necessitate continuous medical attention due to their heightened susceptibility to a range of complications. The primary portion of healthcare costs related to diabetes is allocated to complications such as cardiovascular disease, which can be significantly prevented by avoiding the development of issues (Howse et al., 2020). Multiple reports indicate that implementing aggressive diabetes control can effectively reduce medical expenses without compromising the standard of care. In order to effectively and cost-efficiently manage diabetes, it is crucial to prevent complications, promptly begin treatment through vigilant monitoring of blood glucose levels, offer proactive education on nutrition and physical activity, and regularly monitor the condition. Moreover, the timely identification of diabetes in its initial stages and the implementation of proactive treatment substantially reduce the occurrence and cost of chronic complications.

Widespread adoption of U-healthcare could potentially result in annual savings of over 457 million USD for the United States. Although U-healthcare is not a substitute for in-person consultation and treatment, it can be highly beneficial in managing chronic conditions such as diabetes mellitus (Howse et al., 2020). Patients diagnosed with diabetes mellitus would experience significant advantages from implementing a telemonitoring or tele coaching strategy for their treatment. This approach would involve maintaining regular hospital visits while managing their health at home through the use of affordable electronic devices. By doing so, patients would stay in constant communication with their physicians and receive medical assistance whenever necessary.

Well-established clinical guidelines govern the management and treatment of diabetes. Nurses can be entrusted with the responsibility of managing prescriptions and providing guidance on lifestyle-related health practices, such as diet and exercise, while maintaining the highest level of care. It is imperative to implement personalized treatment approaches that prioritize prevention and management rather than therapy. Additionally, ensuring patient adherence to chronic illness management is of utmost importance (Howse et al., 2020). The concept underlying "humanistic" or "whole-person" treatment is that frequent engagement with a readily available team of professionals, such as doctors, nurses, dietitians, fitness specialists, and experts in relevant areas, enhances psychological well-being. Collaboration improves the process of monitoring and instruction. Regular communication and information access between the hospital and the patient's home are vital. The patient is capable of consistently providing updates regarding their health.

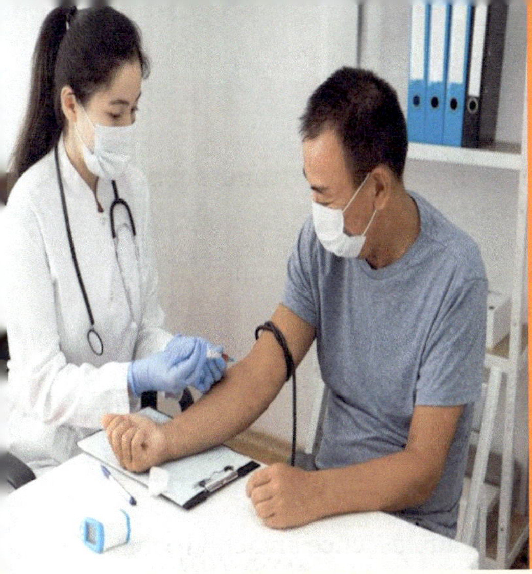

Chapter 8

HEALTH PROMOTION FOR SPECIAL POPULATIONS

Contents

Special populations consist of individuals who may be at a higher risk for long-term illness, exposure to hazardous drugs, or natural disasters. This increased vulnerability can be attributed to various factors such as age, gender, occupation, or behavior. Special populations often include pregnant women, elderly individuals, and children. Additionally, individuals who may fall into this category are those from low-income families, encompassing both adults and children who come from economically disadvantaged backgrounds.

8.1. Children and Adolescents

During childhood and adolescence, significant development occurs in the realms of physical, cognitive, and social growth. There are several important developmental needs that must be addressed during this period. The development of these youth is greatly influenced by parents/guardians, school communities, friends, and society. The presence or absence of positive support and healthy influences can have significant long-term consequences. Throughout life experiences, individuals have the opportunity to develop and grow their capabilities, confidence, and capacities. These processes occur during both childhood and adolescence (Selmani et al., 2021). In some cases, the development of a young person can be negatively impacted by conflict, trauma, or other life events. These situations may necessitate the involvement of helping professionals who can provide interventions and additional support. This stage of development is filled with potential and optimism, yet it can also be quite intricate.

8.1.1. Preventive Measures

Healthy conduct can be instilled and nurtured in children and adolescents through the support of loving families, engaged community members, and friends. When working with young individuals, it is crucial for counselors to possess a comprehensive understanding of the various factors that can influence their behavior. By being well-versed in common risk and protective variables, counselors can effectively guide youth towards making positive choices.

There are various factors that can contribute to both the risk and protection of individuals, including psychological, biological, familial, social, and cultural features. Certain attributes are predetermined, like personality traits or genetic predisposition, while others are subject to change and may fluctuate over time, such as income level or self-esteem.

Risk factors, as defined by the Substance Abuse and Mental Health Services Administration (SAMHSA), are characteristics at various levels – biological, psychological, family, social, community, or cultural – that are often associated with an increased likelihood of negative life outcomes (Selmani et al., 2021).

During the stages of adolescence and childhood, it is imperative to recognize the significance of this period in terms of development and growth. To promote children's and teenager's healthy development, parents and educators can take action both at home and at school. It is important to provide children with consistent and nurturing care, encourage reading, support their academic pursuits, prioritize their sleep, and motivate them to participate in physical activities (Selmani et al., 2021). Health care practitioners have the ability to closely monitor children's behavioral, mental, emotional, and physical development through screenings and other preventive care services. It is crucial to identify issues at an early stage to ensure that children and adolescents receive the necessary developmental support.

Students who are frequently absent from class are at a higher risk of experiencing lower academic performance and facing health issues in the future. In middle school, chronic absence rates tend to start increasing. The reduction of middle school children's absences from school can be achieved through the implementation of community and school-based interventions.

It is recommended to conduct developmental screenings at ages 9, 18, and 24 to 30 months. Healthcare professionals conduct developmental screenings to evaluate a child's abilities in learning, speaking, moving, and socializing. This helps caregivers in identifying developmental issues and giving children the necessary care. One effective approach to increasing the percentage of children receiving developmental screenings is by implementing policies that require healthcare providers to assess children using standardized instruments during routine well-child visits (Selmani et al., 2021).

Many children do not receive an adequate amount of sleep. Insufficient sleep has been linked to the development of diabetes, obesity, and cardiovascular problems. Additionally, it can influence behavior, mood, learning, and concentration. Implementing later school start times, providing parent education, and utilizing behavioral interventions are effective strategies to ensure that children receive adequate sleep.

It is important to note that promoting positive communication between children and adolescents and their parents can have significant health benefits. Discussing beliefs, experiences, and feelings is an essential aspect of effective communication between parents and children. Effective communication is crucial for fostering healthy relationships and ensuring the well-being of children. It has been found to play a significant role in protecting children from health hazards and enhancing their academic performance (Selmani et al., 2021). Improving the quality of communication between parents and children, particularly in cases where behavioral issues are present, can be achieved through family interventions and behavioral parenting strategies.

8.2. Older Adults

Unhealthy habits and lifestyle choices can lead to the development of diseases over time. Investing in health prevention is significantly more cost-effective compared to the expenses incurred when treating an illness. Many older individuals have begun incorporating behavioral techniques into their lives for additional self-health prevention, management, and even recovery, whether they are aware of it or not.

In recent years, the WHO has emphasized the importance of health promotion as the most effective way to improve human health. According to the WHO's vital key facts, the world's population over 60 years of age is projected to reach 22% by 2050. Additionally, it is predicted that by 2030, there will be a greater number of individuals over 60 than children under the age of five (Miller & Iris, 2002). During a meeting of the UN General Assembly, it was declared that the years 2021–2030 will be designated as the UN Decade of Healthy Ageing. This is an important period where the promotion of healthy lifestyles among older individuals will be of utmost importance.

The aging population will have a significant impact on various aspects of society, including the economy, education, social development, health and medical care, and welfare. Obesity in older adult patients is associated with a range of conditions, such as type 2 diabetes, hypertension, and cardiovascular disease. Additionally, it has been found to increase morbidity and mortality rates. It is widely believed by experts that obesity is influenced by a range of factors, some of which may be exacerbated by a sedentary lifestyle. Engaging in physical activity has been shown to have numerous benefits for the elderly population. Research has indicated that those who are active tend to have lower rates of depression, dementia, Alzheimer's disease, fractures, falls, and all-cause and cardiovascular mortality. Additionally, individuals experience an enhanced quality of life and improved cognitive performance, as noted by Miller and Iris in 2002.

Chronic diseases are a significant concern for older individuals, and if not properly managed, they can lead to comorbidities that have long-lasting effects on patients and further burden the healthcare systems of the country. It is crucial to emphasize the significance of illness prevention and health promotion for older individuals, considering their considerably greater medical needs compared to other age groups. The primary goals of disease prevention and health promotion for older individuals revolve around minimizing the negative impact of diseases and ensuring the preservation of physical function and independent living.

Health promotion involves taking a proactive approach to health, with a focus on self-actualization. It empowers individuals to actively develop healthy behaviors and enhance their overall well-being. It is generally not advisable for individuals over the age of 85 to rely heavily on medical assistance from doctors and paramedics. Engaging in regular exercise, giving up smoking, moderating alcohol consumption, and actively participating in social and educational activities are all key components of a healthy lifestyle for older individuals. Some medical professionals strongly believe that embracing a healthy lifestyle can have a greater impact on the health of older individuals compared to relying solely on medication. According to Miller and Iris (2002), a harmful lifestyle is characterized by engaging in unhealthy activities. Engaging in conduct that affects one's own health, whether positively or negatively, is referred to as practicing health behavior. Positive health behaviors encompass activities such as regular exercise and maintaining a well-balanced diet. On the other hand, harmful behaviors encompass smoking, excessive drinking, and engaging in risky sexual activity. Health promotion involves enhancing an individual's overall well-being by implementing various strategies, creating supportive environments, and fostering positive circumstances that contribute to their longevity, mental resilience, and overall quality of life.

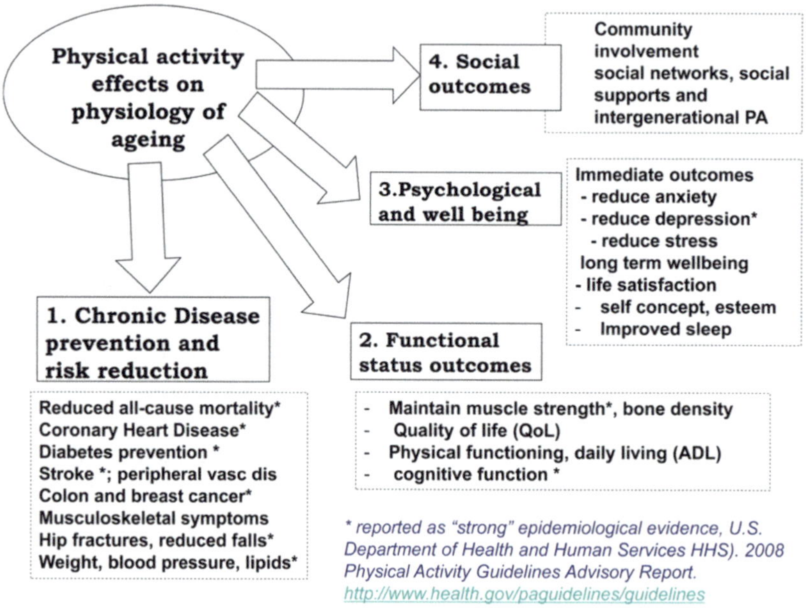

Figure 8.1. *A conceptual framework for the benefits of physical activity in older adults.*

Source: Bauman et al. (2016).

Reducing sedentary behavior and increasing physical exercise in older adults can have a significant impact on their quality of life, stress levels, and physical function. It is important for the general public to understand that exercise treatments not only aim to enhance health, but can also be complemented by the use of technology. Individuals have the ability to perceive their own exercise volume and intensity during physical activity as demonstrated by Miller and Iris in their study conducted in 2002. The novel typology of the exercise and technology combination is primarily focused on the exercise field, as it is the most effective way to achieve maximum workout results (Figure 8.1).

8.3. Women's Health

Women encounter a range of unique health challenges, including menopause, childbirth, and pregnancy. In addition, there are certain health issues that affect both men and women, but women may face unique challenges in dealing with them. Women may experience significant long-term health complications as a result of pregnancy and childbirth. It is crucial to address unintended pregnancies and provide comprehensive care during pregnancy, childbirth, and the postpartum period in order to minimize health complications and mortality rates (Rodin & Ickovics, 1990).

Screening plays a crucial role in identifying and addressing health issues that affect women disproportionately. By conducting regular screenings, we can effectively detect and treat diseases and conditions that are more common among women.

Here are a few strategies for improving women's health:

8.3.1. Reduce Iron Deficiency Among Females Aged 12 to 49 Years

Iron plays a crucial role in facilitating the transportation of oxygen by the blood throughout the entire body. However, it is worth noting that not everyone possesses an adequate amount of this essential element. Women are more susceptible to iron deficiency because they experience blood loss during their menstrual cycles. Another cause of iron deficiency is childbirth and pregnancy. One effective approach to ensuring women receive adequate iron is through the consumption of iron-fortified foods and supplements, as suggested by Rodin and Ickovics (1990). It is highly recommended that individuals utilize the Nutrition Facts label to keep track of their iron consumption (Figure 8.2).

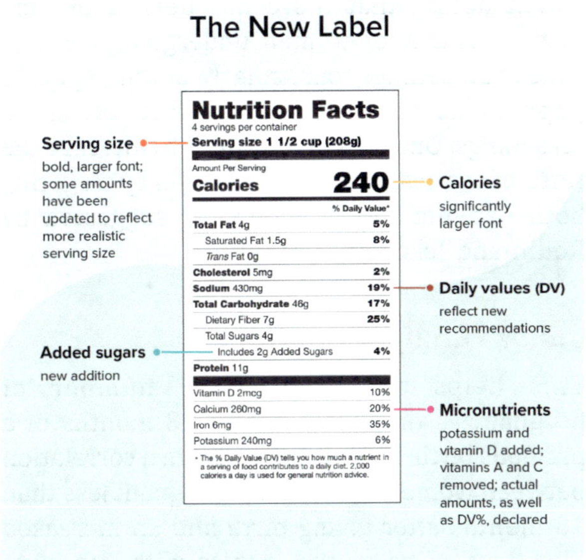

Figure 8.2. *New nutrition facts label.*

Source: Seit (2020).

8.3.2. Reduce the Female Breast and Cervical Cancer Death Rate

Breast cancer is a highly common type of cancer that affects many women in the United States. Although there has been a decline in the fatality rate from breast cancer in recent years, it remains higher in specific racial and ethnic groups. In order to effectively reduce breast cancer deaths, it is crucial to implement community-based cancer control initiatives, develop personalized treatment plans, and enhance screening efforts for this disease (Rodin & Ickovics, 1990). Early detection of breast cancer is crucial in saving women's lives from this devastating disease. It is crucial for women to undergo regular check-ups to reduce the risk of developing breast cancer, ensure early detection, and improve their chances of survival. In order to effectively reduce breast cancer fatalities, it is crucial to enhance the frequency of breast cancer screenings.

Thanks to the Pap test, the risk of developing cervical cancer and mortality rates among women have significantly decreased. It is worth noting that there has been a decline in the number of women undergoing cervical cancer screenings, particularly among specific populations who are less inclined to seek these screenings. One effective strategy to increase the rates of cervical cancer screening is by targeting both patients and providers, as suggested by Rodin and Ickovics in 1990.

8.3.3. Family Planning

This helps to decrease the number of pregnancies that occur within 18 months of a previous birth. Research has shown a correlation between women who become pregnant less than 18 months after giving birth and an increased likelihood of premature babies with low birth weights (Rodin & Ickovics, 1990). In addition, it is important to note that these pregnancies have a higher likelihood of being unplanned, which can lead to additional health concerns for both the woman and the unborn child. One potential approach to increasing the time between pregnancies is by implementing interventions that promote the utilization of birth control and family planning services among women who have recently given birth.

Research has shown that there is a higher likelihood of premature births, low birth weights, and unfortunately, infant mortality rates among teenage mothers. Becoming a mother can have a significant impact on the health, educational, and employment prospects of adolescent moms. Although there have been some improvements in reducing teen pregnancy and births, it is important to acknowledge that disparities based on race and ethnicity continue to persist. There is a wealth of evidence demonstrating the effectiveness of various outreach and teaching initiatives in reducing the incidence of teen pregnancies. One of the goals is to enhance the rate of sexually active adolescent females who opt for a highly or reasonably effective method of contraception during their most recent sexual encounter. In addition to refraining from sexual activity, employing hormonal birth control or an intrauterine device (IUD) alongside a condom is the most reliable approach to prevent pregnancy, as stated by Rodin and Ickovics in 1990. Interestingly, it is worth noting that a significant proportion of adolescent females who engage in sexual activity opted not to utilize an IUD or hormonal birth control method during their most recent encounter. Research has shown that when teenagers are provided with comprehensive education on the risks associated with unprotected sex, it can lead to an increase in the adoption of effective birth control methods.

A significant number of women fail to utilize effective birth control methods that are suitable for their needs. Various factors can impact a woman's likelihood of using effective birth control, such as her insurance status, family income, and marital status (Rodin & Ickovics, 1990).

8.4. Men's Health

On average, women tend to outlive men by approximately five years. It is worth noting that there is a higher incidence of HIV, heart disease, lung cancer, and other serious illnesses among males. It is important to note that men face unique health challenges, including prostate cancer, which is not prevalent among women. Understanding the importance of preventive screenings and routine medical treatment for men of all ages is crucial for enhancing men's health. This knowledge can play a significant role in promoting overall well-being and preventing potential health issues (Baker et al., 2014) (Figure 8.3).

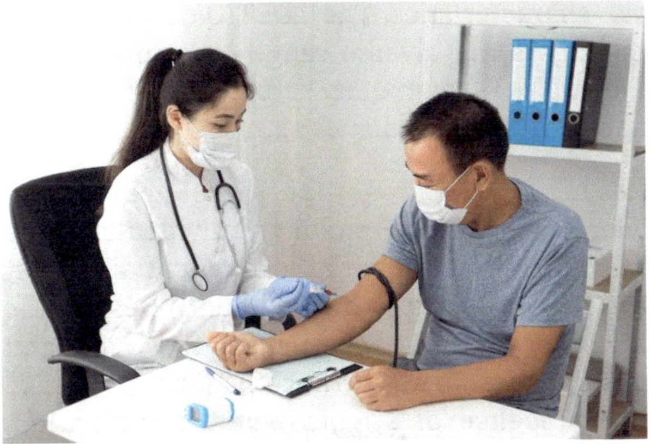

Figure 8.3. *Health screenings for men.*

Source: Blog-Manager (2023).

Improving men's health and preventing diseases can be achieved through the implementation of interventions that discourage drinking and smoking, while promoting healthy habits.

Here are a few strategies for promoting men's health:

- **Reduce the Prostate Cancer Death Rate:** Extensive research has shown that closely monitoring prostate cancer can significantly decrease the mortality rate associated with this disease, particularly in men who receive an early diagnosis. Prostate cancer holds the unfortunate title of being the most frequently diagnosed cancer and the second most common cause of cancer-related deaths in men. There is a significant disparity in prostate cancer death rates among different demographic groups, as highlighted by Baker, et al. in 2014.
- **Increase the Proportion of Sexually Active Adolescent Males Who use a Condom at Last Intercourse:** It is worth noting that a significant portion of new cases of sexually transmitted infections (STIs) reported each year are among adolescents. It is worth noting that a significant number of sexually active teenage males neglected to use a condom in their most recent sexual experience. However, it is crucial to emphasize that condoms play a vital role in the prevention of certain STIs. According to research conducted by Baker, et al., in 2014, the provision of condoms has been found to potentially increase the frequency of teenagers using them.
- **Reduce the Rate of Primary and Secondary Syphilis in Men Who Have Sex with Men:** It is important to note that individuals who engage in sexual activity with other individuals of the same gender have a higher risk of contracting syphilis compared to other demographic groups. It is important to note that untreated syphilis can have serious consequences. Not only does it increase the risk of contracting and spreading HIV, but it can also lead to complications involving the brain and eyes (Baker et al., 2014). Lowering syphilis rates can be achieved through the implementation of preventive measures such as condom usage, regular screening, and prompt treatment for both the infected individual and their sexual partner.
- **Reduce Gonorrhea Rates Among Adolescent and Young Males:** There has been a recent increase in the prevalence of gonorrhea, specifically among

men. Furthermore, the contraction of gonorrhea can lead to the development of pelvic inflammatory disease in women, in addition to increasing the risk of HIV infection and transmission. In the near future, it is possible for gonorrhea to develop resistance to the last recommended medication, as mentioned by Baker, et al. (2014). Ensuring the prevention of untreated gonorrhea and reducing the chances of incurable infections heavily rely on the screening of individuals at high risk and promptly starting treatment following diagnosis.

It is worth noting that there is a significant disparity in the number of doctor visits between men and women. Specifically, men attend doctors' offices 150 million fewer times each year compared to women. Regrettably, the decreased figure fails to accurately represent the overall health of both men and women. It is a common observation that men often tend to neglect seeking medical attention when they are unwell or dealing with a health condition that necessitates care (Baker et al., 2014). What is the reason for their refusal to depart? There are multiple possible explanations for this, and here are a few examples:

- Disliking unfavorable information
- Examination discomfort
- Apprehension of appearing weak

8.5. LGBTQ+ Health

LGBTIQ+ health encompasses the overall well-being of individuals who identify as lesbian, gay, bisexual, transgender, intersex, or queer, encompassing their mental, emotional, and physical health. Sexual Orientation, Gender Identity and Expression, and Sex Characteristics (SOGIESC) represents the vast range of human diversity when it comes to sexual orientation, gender identity, expression, and sex characteristics. The LGBTIQ+ abbreviation highlights the diverse range of groups within the LGBTIQ+ community across different nations and locations (Taylor et al., 2013).

Research indicates that there are certain shared experiences among individuals in the LGBTIQ+ community that can potentially affect their overall health and well-being. Despite the diversity within this community, these common experiences are worth considering. Due to the presence of stigma and discrimination, individuals may be less inclined to engage with healthcare professionals and access necessary treatments, resulting in detrimental effects on their overall physical and emotional well-being. They may also experience human rights violations, including acts of violence, torture, criminalization, forced medical treatment, and discrimination. In healthcare settings, patients may unfortunately encounter incorrect pathologizing, discriminatory attitudes, and denial of care based on their SOGIESC (Taylor et al., 2013).

One of the fundamental principles of human rights is the belief that every individual should have equal access to healthcare. This principle serves as the foundation for the World Health Organization's support to nations. Understanding and improving the health and well-being of LGBTIQ+ individuals has been highlighted by the adoption of the 2030 Agenda for Sustainable Development and its commitment to inclusivity, drawing on the principles of international human rights law. For the purpose of aiding nations in the development and strengthening of comprehensive health systems and policies that prioritize the health and well-being of all individuals, irrespective of their sexual orientation, gender identity, gender expression, or sex characteristics, the WHO provides guidelines, technical support, and conducts research (Taylor et al., 2013).

Healthcare providers who specialize in LGBTQ+ care have identified the following health issues as commonly concerning for transgender individuals. It is important to note that not all of these items are applicable to every individual. However, it is advisable to have an understanding of these matters.

8.5.1. Access to Healthcare

Locating a medical professional with the necessary qualifications to provide care for transgender patients can be a complex task, even though there has been some improvement in recent years. It is crucial for transgender patients to seek out a primary care physician who not only embraces their identity but also possesses the essential training and experience to provide them with the appropriate treatment they need. There may be instances where your insurance company will not cover the expenses of therapy, even if you are able to locate a provider (Taylor et al., 2013). It is important to refer to your insurance policy in order to determine if your expenses will be covered. Consider discussing alternative options for affordable treatment with your healthcare provider if the costs are not included.

8.5.2. Conditions Related to the Heart

Transgender individuals may face an increased risk of heart attacks and strokes due to factors such as smoking, being overweight, having high blood pressure, and having diabetes. It is important to note that transgender women may choose not to discuss certain symptoms, such as breathing difficulties or chest pain, out of concern that their physician may advise them to discontinue estrogen if they have heart issues (Taylor et al., 2013). It is important to promptly notify your physician if you encounter any of these symptoms.

8.5.3. HIV and Other STIs

In recent years, there has been a significant increase in the ability to prevent the acquisition and transmission of HIV. Anti-HIV drugs have the remarkable ability to enable individuals living with HIV to lead normal lives and significantly decrease the chances of transmitting the virus to their sexual partners. This approach, known as Treatment and Prevention, not only provides peace of mind but also eliminates the anxiety often associated with engaging in sexual activities. According to research findings, it has been established that engaging in intercourse while taking anti-HIV drugs and maintaining an undetectable viral level renders the transmission of HIV impossible (undetectable equals untransmittable).

Pre-exposure prophylaxis, also known as PrEP, has proven to be an incredibly effective method for nearly eliminating the risk of HIV infection in individuals who are currently uninfected (Taylor et al., 2013). By promptly initiating post-exposure prophylaxis (PEP) within 72 hours of an unexpected HIV exposure, individuals who are not on PrEP can greatly reduce their chances of acquiring the virus.

8.5.4. Tobacco and Alcohol

Excessive alcohol consumption can have detrimental effects on various organs, including the liver. This level of consumption can also lead to negative behavior towards others or oneself, as well as reckless driving. It has been observed that there is a higher prevalence of smoking among transsexual individuals. It is important to note that individuals who use hormones may be at a higher risk of developing lung and heart problems, as highlighted by Taylor et al. in 2013. It is advisable to consult with your primary care physician regarding your alcohol and tobacco consumption habits. If you are interested in reducing or quitting – don't hesitate to seek assistance.

8.5.5. Depression

Depression is a prevalent issue that affects many individuals within the transgender community due to a range of factors. It is important to note that depression can continue to be present even after a transition. It is important to communicate with your therapist or provider about any feelings of depression or sadness you may be experiencing. This will allow for a discussion about your emotions and how to address them. There are multiple treatment options available for depression.

8.6. Racial and Ethnic Minorities

Racism is a societal construct that evaluates an individual's worth and opportunities solely on the basis of their physical appearance or skin color. This complex system is composed of various institutions, regulations, practices, and conventions. According to Richardson and Norris (2010), there is a clear disparity in society where some individuals are unjustly advantaged while others endure hardships. The detrimental effects of interpersonal and institutional racism are far-reaching, significantly compromising the emotional and physical well-being of countless individuals. These barriers hinder their capacity to achieve optimal health and have a profound impact on the overall health of our nation.

Communities of color have been significantly impacted by the enduring effects of racism in many nations, as supported by a growing body of research. This phenomenon has far-reaching implications that are deeply embedded in our society. It leads to unequal opportunities in areas such as housing, wealth, education, and employment. Additionally, it shapes individuals' choices regarding their residential locations, educational institutions, workplaces, places of worship, and cultural activities (Richardson & Norris, 2010). The circumstances discussed here, commonly known as social determinants of health, play a significant role in creating health disparities within communities of color. These factors significantly raise the likelihood of negative health outcomes for individuals belonging to these communities.

Health inequality can be observed in various ways. One significant factor is the presence of structural or institutional racism, which manifests in laws, regulations, and social practices that favor certain racial groups over others. One example of the detrimental impact of systemic racism in the criminal justice system is the negative health effects it can have. Various means, such as language, attitudes, media, and symbols, are employed to perpetuate the notion of inferiority among certain populations. This phenomenon is commonly referred to as cultural racism. One example of how racial preconceptions can impact housing preferences is the potential for racial segregation in neighborhoods among White property owners. According to Richardson and Norris (2010), the presence of unfavorable housing and environmental conditions can lead to the formation of communities characterized by concentrated poverty.

Individual-level discrimination refers to the occurrence of intentional or inadvertent prejudice against racial groups by individuals or organizations. This could potentially lead to limited access to employment opportunities, education, and healthcare.

Experiencing racism has been found to have a significant impact on both mental and, to a lesser degree, physical well-being. Multiple studies have provided evidence suggesting that the physical and mental toll of experiencing racism can have lasting effects on one's health. Stress can have a significant impact on our long-term health, as it weakens our immune system and raises blood pressure. Racism has been linked to elevated stress levels, resulting in a higher likelihood of developing high blood pressure among individuals from marginalized communities (Richardson & Norris, 2010). According to the CDC Trusted Source, research indicates that hypertension is more prevalent among black individuals compared to other racial or ethnic groups.

In a study conducted in 2019, it was found that exposure to racism among African Americans has been linked to increased inflammation. This, in turn, raises their susceptibility to chronic illnesses such as kidney and heart disease (Richardson & Norris, 2010). A recent study has revealed that the unfair treatment of individuals from marginalized communities can have a significant impact on their sleep patterns and overall physiological well-being during midlife.

Extensive research has established a clear correlation between structural racism within the medical system and its detrimental impact on physical health. As an example, a study conducted in 2016 examined the relationship between racial bias and pain management. The study found that incorrect biological assumptions, such as the belief that "Black people's skin is thicker than White people's skin," were associated with the undertreatment of pain in Black patients.

Based on credible research, it has been found that there is a disparity in the prescription of medication for Black children experiencing severe appendicitis pain compared to children from other racial backgrounds. According to Richardson and Norris (2010), it has been observed that medical personnel may unintentionally or intentionally use different pain thresholds for different racial groups when providing care, potentially due to racial bias.

8.7. Individuals with Disabilities

According to Harrison (2006), approximately 1.3 billion people are believed to experience significant impairment. Approximately 1 in 6 individuals, which is equivalent to 16% of the world's population, falls into this category. It has been observed that individuals with disabilities may experience a significantly shorter lifespan compared to those without disabilities, with some passing away as much as two decades earlier. People with impairments have a higher likelihood of developing various health conditions, including obesity, diabetes, asthma, depression, and poor dental health. People with impairments are impacted by various health disparities.

According to Harrison (2006), individuals with impairments face significantly greater challenges in accessing affordable transportation compared to those without disabilities. The root cause of health disparities lies in the unfair situations that individuals with disabilities are forced to confront. These situations encompass stigma, discrimination, poverty, exclusion from school and work, and various obstacles within the healthcare system.

People with impairments have a higher likelihood of experiencing premature mortality, poorer overall health, and greater challenges in their daily activities.

There are several factors that contribute to health inequities for individuals with disabilities:

- **The Existence of Unjust Conditions Which Contributes to the Emergence of Health Inequalities: Factors of Structure:** People with disabilities face significant challenges in various aspects of life, including stigma, discrimination, and ableism. These factors have a profound effect on their overall mental and physical well-being. Freedom of choice can sometimes be limited by laws and policies, which can unfortunately support certain harmful medical procedures such as forced sterilization, involuntary admission and treatment, and even institutionalization (Harrison, 2006).

- **Social Determinants of Health:** Individuals with disabilities are at a higher risk of facing health challenges and not having their healthcare needs met when they live in poor conditions, face poverty, and are excluded from educational and employment opportunities. Individuals with disabilities often rely on the support of their families in order to engage in various health and community activities, as there are often limitations in the available social support systems. According to Harrison (2006), this situation has negative consequences for both individuals with disabilities and their caregivers, who are predominantly women and girls.
- **Risk Factors:** Non-communicable disease risk factors (e.g., smoking, poor diet, excessive alcohol consumption, and lack of exercise) are more prevalent among individuals with disabilities. Exclusion from public health programs is a significant contributing factor, as highlighted by Harrison (2006).
- **Health System:** The health system presents numerous challenges for individuals with disabilities across all aspects. One of the main reasons behind the health disparities experienced by this group is the insufficient dissemination of information, negative attitudes, and discriminatory behavior exhibited by healthcare professionals. Additionally, the lack of accessibility to healthcare facilities and information further exacerbates the issue. Furthermore, the absence of comprehensive data collection and analysis specifically focusing on disabilities contributes to the problem.

For the achievement of health for all, it is crucial to prioritize disability inclusion as it aligns with global health priorities and the Sustainable Development Goals. In order to achieve universal health coverage, it is imperative that individuals with disabilities receive equitable treatment and access to top-notch healthcare services. Failure to address this issue will hinder the realization of universal health coverage. Communities stand to benefit greatly from the implementation of universal health care, which would provide much-needed support for both individuals with impairments and the general population. Implementing disability inclusive prevention and care for noncommunicable illnesses could potentially result in a significant return on investment. According to Harrison (2006), for every dollar invested, there could be a nearly tenfold return.

It is crucial to consider the needs of individuals with disabilities when addressing and preparing for health emergencies, as they are more susceptible to both direct and indirect impacts. As a consequence of the COVID-19 pandemic, individuals with disabilities living in institutions have experienced a significant disconnection from the broader society. There have been reports of inmates being excessively medicated, subjected to drug use, or confined, along with cases of self-inflicted harm. During the COVID-19 pandemic, it was observed that individuals with intellectual disabilities faced higher fatality rates and had a lower likelihood of needing critical care.

In order to effectively address and prevent issues such as road safety, clean air and water, child nutrition, and violence against women, it is crucial to consider the needs, abilities, and talents of individuals with disabilities. By taking these factors into account, we can work towards promoting healthier populations. According to Harrison (2006), research shows that women with disabilities are 2.4 times more likely to experience intimate partner violence compared to non-disabled women (Figure 8.4).

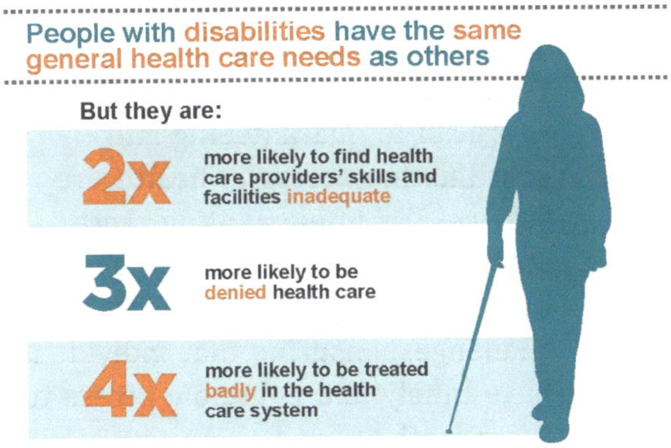

Figure 8.4. *People with disabilities continue to be underserved by health systems.*

Source: Miller (2021).

8.8. Rural Health Promotion

There are a multitude of factors that have an impact on the health of rural communities. In rural populations, chronic conditions are more prevalent when compared to their urban counterparts. Chronic ailments encompass a range of conditions, including heart disease, cancer, chronic respiratory diseases, strokes, and diabetes. When we compare rural areas to metropolitan communities, we find that mortality and disability rates tend to be higher in the former (Goeppinger, 1993). These health issues are worsened by the lack of access to healthcare services, programs, and initiatives aimed at preventing diseases and promoting good health.

Here are a few examples of societal factors that hinder the provision of healthcare in rural areas:

- Higher rates of poverty.
- Social and cultural standards related to healthy behavior.
- Limited understanding of health and incomplete health beliefs.
- Differences in education and language.
- Limited access to affordable, reliable, or public transportation.
- Unpredictable work schedules or unemployment.
- Decreased population densities to ensure cost-effective program coverage.
- Limited resources that can assist staff members, facilitate the use of facilities, and streamline program administration.
- Limited options when it comes to engaging in physical activity and consuming healthy food.

Rural programs face numerous challenges such as poverty, chronic illness, low educational attainment, and limited transportation access. However, they have the potential to implement impactful health promotion and disease prevention initiatives. In order for programs to achieve success in promoting health, it is crucial for them to acknowledge and make the most of the assets within the community. According to Goeppinger (1993), these advantages have the potential to help rural areas overcome obstacles when it comes to implementing disease prevention and health promotion programs. Some of the benefits of living in rural areas include:

- Having strong social networks and connections for the well-being of individuals and communities.
- Maintaining ties with neighbors and family members, as these relationships contribute to the upliftment of societies.
- People share similar ideals and have a collective desire to enhance health, hence positive changes can be made.
- Developing programs with a smaller scope and size, which can potentially accelerate opportunities.
- Demonstrating the courage and willingness to confront obstacles.
- Implementing centralized routes for communication.
- Emphasizing originality and a strong dedication to achieving success.

When developing population health strategies in rural areas, it is important to consider several key factors:

- **Socioeconomic Determinants of Health Within the Community:** This will provide valuable insights into the unique challenges and needs of the population.
- **Involving the Community in the Planning and Implementation Process:** This is essential for fostering a sense of ownership and ensuring that strategies are tailored to their specific needs.
- **Building Alliances and Promoting Teamwork Among Various Stakeholders:** This is vital for the success of population health initiatives. By working together, organizations and individuals can leverage their strengths and resources to address health disparities effectively. It is also important to acknowledge the advantages, disadvantages, difficulties, and obstacles that may arise when implementing population health strategies in rural areas. By recognizing these factors, healthcare providers and policymakers can develop proactive solutions and mitigate potential barriers.
- **Utilizing Integrated Services, Transportation, and Care Coordination Techniques:** This is crucial to guaranteeing and coordinating access to healthcare services. By implementing these strategies, rural communities can overcome geographical and logistical challenges, ensuring that individuals have timely and equitable access to the care they need.

8.8.1. Strategies for Enhancing Health in Rural Areas

8.8.1.1. Health Communication

This is a crucial field that plays a vital role in promoting public health. It involves the dissemination of information and messages related to health issues, with the aim of raising awareness and influencing behavior change. Effective health communication requires clear and concise messaging, tailored to different target audiences. By employing various communication channels. Health communication techniques encompass both written and spoken forms of communication, with the goal of empowering and persuading individuals, groups, and communities to make healthier decisions (Goeppinger, 1993). In order to foster positive changes in attitudes and behaviors, health communication often incorporates various theories and models. Social marketing (involving the development of programs and initiatives to promote positive behavior change) is closely linked to health communication.

Health-related messages have the power to shape campaigns at various levels, including community, small-group, interpersonal, and mass media. This is achieved by utilizing a diverse range of communication channels. Health communication tactics aim to modify individuals' beliefs, practices, and/or knowledge. Here are a few examples of these efforts:

- Enhance the perception of risk
- Promote positive behavior
- Influence societal norms
- Increase access to essential services and support
- Empower individuals to modify or improve their health situations

8.8.1.2. Health Education

This provides individuals with the necessary information, skills, and resources to enhance their quality of life. It offers a range of learning experiences focused on various health-related topics. Health education strategies are tailored to suit the specific needs of the target population, as discussed by Goeppinger in 1993. Health education provides individuals with valuable information on a range of health topics, including the benefits and potential risks to their well-being. It also offers resources to support individuals in making positive changes to their behavior within a conducive environment and building their capacity.

One can offer education on population, community, and individual health. There are several examples of health education initiatives at these three levels:

- **At the Individual Level**
    - At the individual level, there is a focus on personal communication and interaction.
- **At the Local Level**
    - There are lectures that aim to impart fundamental knowledge to small groups.
    - Workshops are conducted to facilitate a series of meetings where small groups can engage in discussions about the topic(s).
    - Panel or group discussions can be organized to encourage interactive dialog on the topic.
    - Webinars can be conducted to provide real-time access to information.
- **At the Population Level**
    - It is important to take into account TV shows or commercials that are intended for a wide audience.
    - There are advertisements or radio shows that are specifically designed to target listeners with particular tastes.
    - Consider utilizing a newspaper or other printed materials as a means of effectively conveying specific details.
    - Utilizing social media platforms to disseminate captivating images.

8.9. Immigrant Health Promotion

The Refugee Health Promotion (RHP) Program provides financial support to grantees who offer direct services to promote the health and well-being of refugees. These services are provided on a regular basis and are also available during times of emergency, such as a pandemic.

The three primary goals of RHP are:

i. Offer chances to improve health literacy;
ii. Organize the medical and psychological care; and
iii. Form health groupings.

Activities and services funded by RHP may include health awareness programs and individual health outreach initiatives.

Another valuable resource for individuals seeking support is peer support meetings, skill-building networks, or adjustment groups specifically designed for medical and mental health purposes.

Services and activities funded by RHP may be included are health education classes, targeted health outreach to individuals, assistance with medical and mental health navigation, support in building skills, adjustment groups, and peer support meetings. RHP services are provided to individuals who meet the requirements for ORR-funded services for a maximum of five years. Grantees are advised to prioritize those with the most ongoing, urgent, or underserved health needs (Hyman & Guruge, 2002).

Understanding the perspectives of refugees and migrants is crucial for effective health promotion practices, as it allows us to recognize the minor organizational and cultural distinctions between ethnic groups that can have a significant impact.

Migrants and refugees face a range of challenges, such as financial constraints, legal and human rights limitations, language barriers, and cultural and religious differences. Limited access to social services and health care can have a detrimental impact on individuals, leading to increased social isolation and potential health risks (Hyman & Guruge, 2002). To empower individuals and enhance their autonomy in managing their life and health, it is the duty of the health promoter to offer support in training, resource allocation, and education. It would be beneficial for them to engage in partnerships with organizations that provide assistance to refugees and migrants.

The primary objective of raising awareness is to establish a connection between refugees and migrants and the essential services they require, achieved through the distribution of current and relevant information. The material is distributed to the intended audience, which includes health professionals, migrants, and refugees, using appropriate communication channels. According to Hyman and Guruge (2002), engaging in face-to-face interactions with peer educators or medical professionals can prove to be an effective strategy. Various channels of communication play a crucial role in spreading knowledge and developing relevant skills. These include social media, mainstream media, as well as resources such as pamphlets and regional language movies. Health promotion plays a crucial role in educating refugees and migrants about their rights, the healthcare resources available to them, and other important information.

In order to effectively promote health among refugees and migrants, it is crucial to ensure the seamless functioning of a network of community-based organizations. However, it is important to note that in many countries, there exist non-governmental organizations, volunteer groups, and social clubs that provide assistance to refugees and migrants. The government has a crucial role in enhancing networks that are currently lacking or underperforming due to capacity constraints. This can be achieved by providing community-based organizations with the essential funding and training they need. Government assistance for the growth and capacity building of non-governmental organizations that assist refugees and migrants is an important policy option (Hyman & Guruge, 2002). It is of utmost importance for government and third-sector organizations to establish connections with refugee and migrant communities, especially those who are most vulnerable to health issues. By leveraging social networks and fostering collaborations, refugees and migrants have the opportunity to play an active role in shaping the development of health services and influencing the way society engages with them.

Migration can lead to a variety of challenges, including heightened exposure to infectious diseases, violence, drug and alcohol abuse, and psychosocial issues. Consequently, the well-being of migrants and refugees may be significantly affected in terms of their reproductive, mental, and sexual health. It is crucial to prioritize the provision of a culturally responsive health promotion service that can effectively address the most critical issues and maximize the potential for improving health outcomes. Health promotion plays a crucial role in enhancing the understanding of refugees and migrants regarding the promotion of health and wellbeing (Hyman & Guruge, 2002). When examining the best practices for health promotion among refugees and migrants, it becomes evident that interventions that are culturally aware and tailored to their specific needs have proven to be more effective than relying solely on mainstream methods.

When it comes to selecting tailored health promotion initiatives, one important aspect is collaborating with community-based organizations. This collaboration can help in offering screening and immunization services, along with peer education to promote the importance of condom usage. There is some conflicting data regarding the effectiveness of health literacy, but collaborating with refugees and migrants to develop this strategy could potentially enhance its efficacy (Hyman & Guruge, 2002). In addition to print materials, videos, and social media, it can be beneficial to ensure that the language used is appropriate and that the content is reinforced through interpersonal or small group interactions.

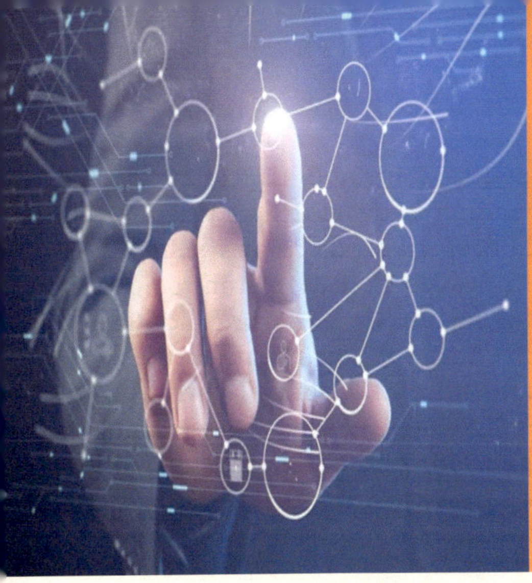

Chapter 9
GLOBAL HEALTH PROMOTION

Contents

9.1. Global Burden of Disease

Over the next 20 years, there will be significant changes in the health demands of the global population. A significant majority of the global population resides in developing nations, where noncommunicable disorders like depression and heart disease are rapidly surpassing traditional causes of disability and premature mortality, such as hunger and infectious diseases. By 2030, it is projected that noncommunicable diseases will account for 70% of deaths in emerging nations, a significant increase from the current rate of less than 50%. It is worth noting that the prevalence of unintentional and intentional injuries is on the rise. In fact, there is a possibility that by 2030, these injuries could surpass infectious diseases as the primary cause of illness worldwide (Murray & Lopez, 2013). These effects are expected to be induced by the aging of the population in developing countries. When the birth rate declines and the proportion of adults to children rises, there is a shift in the most common health issues within a population. These health issues transition from being primarily associated with children to becoming more prevalent among adults. It is worth noting that the "epidemiological transition" has made significant progress in China, various Asian countries, and Latin America (which may not be fully recognized by many public health experts) (Murray & Lopez, 2013). The rapid pace of change and the large number of individuals involved will present considerable challenges for health care systems in general, leading to difficult decisions regarding the allocation of limited resources. Until now, many governments have lacked access to essential information needed for informed discussions and setting public health priorities (Figure 9.1).

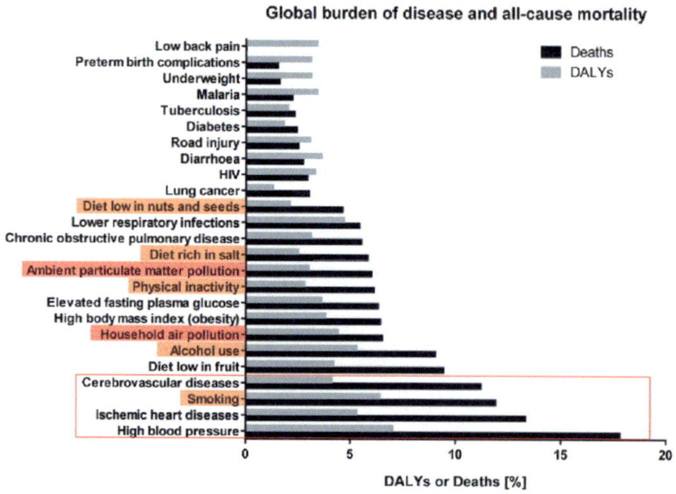

Figure 9.1. *Global burden of disease and related deaths.*

Source: Daiber et al. (2019).

9.1.1. The Current State of the World's Mortality Rate

Many developing nations continue to lack a comprehensive understanding of the factors contributing to population mortality. One of the main objectives of the Global Burden of Disease has been to create comprehensive and internally consistent estimates of the global death toll from each major cause in 1990 (Murray & Lopez, 2013). Prior to the establishment of the Global Burden of Disease, there was a notable absence of any available data set.

The death toll is organized using a hierarchical structure.

At the first level of disaggregation, we can identify three broad cause groups.

- Group 1 focuses on communicable, maternal, perinatal, and nutritional problems.
- Group 2 focuses on noncommunicable diseases.
- Group 3 focuses on injuries.

Despite the ongoing epidemiological change, the impact of infectious disease-related fatalities, perinatal and maternal illnesses, and nutritional deficiencies on society remains significant and largely preventable. Over the past three decades, efforts to maintain control have been remarkably successful. In 1990, a staggering 17.3 million lives were lost due to this set of causes. Developing nations, particularly Sub-Saharan Africa and India, bore the brunt of this devastating toll, with over 16.5 million deaths occurring in these regions. According to Murray and Lopez (2013), the combination of pneumonia and diarrheal illness was responsible for 40% of the deaths in Group 1, resulting in nearly 7 million fatalities in total. There were over 2.4 million deaths related to prenatal disorders, and an additional 2.0 million deaths were a result of tuberculosis. According to Murray and Lopez (2013), a significant number of these deaths could have been prevented if appropriate measures were in place.

The age distribution of mortality varies significantly across different regions due to the disproportionate impact of Group 1 illnesses on children. It is important to note that in Sub-Saharan Africa, there is a significant probability of 22% that a baby girl born in this region may unfortunately pass away before reaching the age of 15.

Among young individuals, there is a notable concentration of these deaths. In this age range, traffic accidents, suicide, war, fire, and violence have been identified as some of the leading causes of death.

9.2. Health Inequalities

Extensive research has shown that various social factors, including education, employment status, income level, gender, and ethnicity, have a profound impact on an individual's overall health. It is important to note that the health of different social groups varies significantly across nations, regardless of their income level. One important factor to consider is the correlation between an individual's socioeconomic status and their risk of experiencing poor health. It has been observed that as socioeconomic status decreases, the likelihood of encountering health issues tends to rise. It is important to consider the impact of socioeconomic circumstances on people's health status and the distribution of health resources across different demographic groups (Scambler, 2012). Health inequalities refer to the disparities that exist in healthcare. Reducing unfair health disparities requires a thoughtful combination of governmental initiatives.

There is often a strong connection between the broader factors of health. As an example, individuals who are unemployed may find themselves living in inadequate housing with limited opportunities to enjoy nature and access nutritious food. It is evident that specific populations and groups are more prone to experiencing poorer health compared to the general population. Certain populations may face challenges when it comes to accessing healthcare, as highlighted by Scambler (2012).

There are several intricate factors that contribute to this situation. For instance, factors that individuals may consider when looking for services include the opening hours and availability in their immediate location, transportation options, accessibility to daycare, language proficiency (both written and spoken), literacy levels, past negative experiences, misinformation, and fear.

Those who are most affected by these disparities are individuals living in areas with high levels of privilege, belonging to Black, Asian, and minority ethnic populations, and being part of inclusive health groups such as the homeless. Health disparities, being preventable, go against the principles of social justice. These occurrences do not occur by chance or without purpose. One's social development is greatly influenced by external factors that are largely beyond their personal control. These conditions have a detrimental impact on individuals, diminishing their prospects for a longer and healthier life (Scambler, 2012).

Implementing the most effective strategies to reduce health disparities is crucial at a national scale. It is crucial to actively work towards stopping or modifying policies that have been proven to worsen inequality or have the potential to do so. It is crucial to recognize the important role that national organizations, particularly those in the public and nonprofit sectors, have in promoting local delivery. This is achieved through advocacy and the development of supporting data, as highlighted by Scambler (2012).

9.2.1. Disparities in Healthy Life Expectancy

Understanding the significance of maintaining good health in enhancing one's quality of life and enabling them to engage in activities they enjoy, a crucial measure of health inequality lies in the duration of time individuals experience good health over their lifespans. One commonly used metric is the average life expectancy in good health. This calculation determines the duration of time individuals spend in a state of "good" or "very good" health, based on their personal perceptions and descriptions of their overall well-being (Figure 9.2).

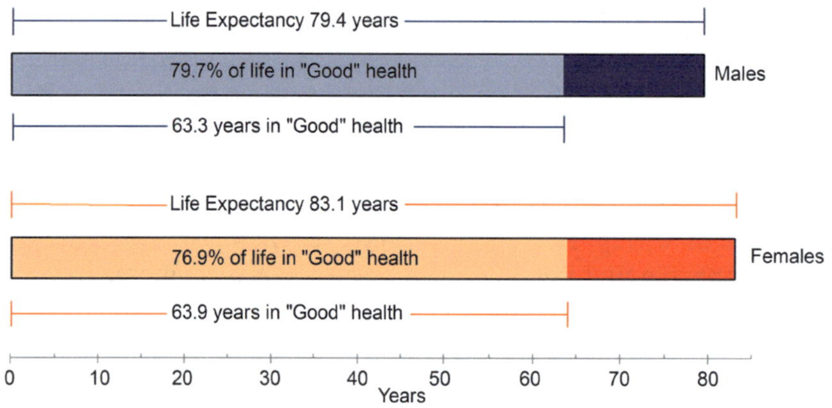

Figure 9.2. *Life expectancy (LE), healthy life expectancy (HLE) and proportion of life in "Good" health for males and females at birth in England, 2011 to 2013.*

Source: Steel (2015).

There is a noticeable discrepancy between the lack of resources and the expected length of a healthy life from the moment of birth. Residents in the least poor areas can expect to enjoy nearly two decades of good health longer than those in the most deprived areas (Scambler, 2012). It is worth noting that individuals residing in the most impoverished regions experience a significantly higher proportion of their lives in a state of poor health compared to those residing in more affluent areas. In fact, this disparity is even more pronounced as the former group spends twice as much time in ill health as the latter. It can be inferred that individuals residing in disadvantaged areas will experience longer periods of illness compared to those in more privileged areas.

9.2.2. Avoidable Mortality Inequalities

Differences in preventable death rates among different demographic groups can be attributed to disparities in access to healthcare for illnesses and dangers that pose a significant risk to their lives. In 2019, there was a significant increase in the likelihood of preventable deaths among women in England's most impoverished districts compared to those in the least deprived areas. Men residing in the most deprived areas faced a significantly higher risk of mortality from preventable causes, with a 3.6-fold increase compared to their counterparts in the least poor areas.

In order to tackle the numerous factors that contribute to health inequities, it is essential to approach the issue with a coordinated, methodical, and persistent effort. These factors encompass a wide range of elements, including variations in healthcare experiences and quality, as well as broader determinants of health. This encompasses the health and care system, but it extends far beyond it. Collaboration across sectors, communities, and services at the local, regional, and federal levels is necessary (Scambler, 2012).

9.3. The Sustainable Development Goals

The path towards a brighter and more sustainable future for all lies within the Sustainable Development Goals. They address global issues such as poverty, inequality, the environment, climate change, peace, and justice. It is absolutely crucial that we achieve all 17 Goals by 2030 in order to ensure that no one is left behind. This is because all of these goals are interconnected (Hák et al., 2016).

9.3.1. The 17 Global Goals

1. No Poverty: Having access to necessities for hygiene, education, and health.
2. Zero Hunger: Establishing sustainable food production, giving food and humanitarian aid.
3. Well-being and Good Health: Enhanced, more easily available health services to prolong life.
4. High-quality education: To promote upward social mobility and eradicate poverty, inclusive education.
5. Gender Equality: Promoting gender-neutral education, advancing laws promoting equality, and ensuring more equitable representation for women.
6. Clean Water and Sanitation: Enhancing accessibility for billions of people who do not have these essential amenities.
7. Accessible and Clean Energy: Ensuring that everyone has access to safe, readily available, and renewable energy sources.
8. Decent Work and Sustainable Economic Growth: Creating jobs for everyone to raise living standards and promote sustainable economic growth.
9. Industry, Innovation, and Infrastructure: Using innovation to create jobs and revenue.
10. Decreased Inequalities: lessening disparities in wealth and other factors both within and between nations.
11. Sustainable Communities and Cities: Creating resilient, safe, and sustainable cities.
12. Responsible Production and Consumption: Countering Present Consumption Patterns and Fostering a Future More Sustainable.

13. Addressing Climate Change: Enforcing regulations, cutting emissions, and advancing renewable energy.
14. Life Below Water: Protecting the Environment, Fostering Marine Biodiversity, and Controlling Fishing Methods.
15. Life on Land: Preserving the environment by reversing human-caused deforestation and desertification.
16. Peace, Justice, and Robust Institutions: Creating inclusive communities with robust institutions and equitable access to justice.
17. Partners for the Goals: Rejuvenate robust international collaborations for sustainable development.

This section will focus specifically on Goal 3 – well-being and good health. Over the past few years, there has been remarkable advancement in improving the overall well-being of individuals. According to Hák, et al. (2016), the SDG objective for under-5 mortality has been achieved or is anticipated to be met by 146 out of 200 nations or regions. From 2010 onwards, there has been a significant decrease of 52% in the number of deaths caused by AIDS-related causes globally, all thanks to the effectiveness of HIV therapy. Additionally, it is worth noting that 47 nations have successfully eliminated at least one neglected tropical illness.

However, it is important to note that there are still disparities in access to healthcare. The progress of Goal 3 development has faced significant obstacles due to the COVID-19 epidemic and various ongoing challenges. When we examine the data, we can observe an alarming increase in the mortality rates due to malaria and tuberculosis...which is concerning. Additionally, there has been a significant decline in childhood vaccination rates, the largest drop we have seen in three decades (Hák et al., 2016).

According to the ambitious Sustainable Development Goals, it is projected that by 2030, AIDS, TB, malaria, and other infectious disease epidemics will be completely eliminated. The objective is to achieve universal health care and provide widespread access to affordable, top-notch medications and vaccinations. Increased funding for health systems is imperative in order to address persistent challenges in healthcare and facilitate the recovery of nations from previous setbacks (Hák et al., 2016). Additionally, this will enhance their ability to withstand potential health hazards in the future.

9.3.2. Access to Essential Health Services

It is a matter of great concern that a significant number of individuals worldwide continue to lack access to vital healthcare services. Addressing discrepancies is crucial in order to close the gap and ensure equal access to healthcare. In order to accomplish the Sustainable Development Goals and work towards our collective objective of Health for All, it is crucial to consider various factors that influence health, including environmental and commercial factors (Hák et al., 2016).

Ensuring a healthy life for everyone requires a substantial commitment, but the benefits outweigh any drawbacks. A strong population is essential for a strong economy. It is imperative that nations across the globe take immediate and decisive action to proactively anticipate and tackle health concerns. It is of utmost importance to consider the well-being of vulnerable populations and individuals residing in regions with a high disease burden. Through this approach, we have the opportunity to enhance health systems and foster resilience in the face of health-related challenges. Vaccination is widely recognized as a highly effective and cost-efficient health intervention on a global scale. It is concerning to note that there has been a significant decline in childhood vaccination rates, which is the largest and most sustained reduction in immunization rates in the past three decades. This decline puts millions of children at risk of preventable diseases that can be fatal.

9.4. International Health Organizations

Various organizations, of varying sizes, contribute to global health assistance. Even for those well-versed in this field, the specific roles carried out by these organizations can sometimes be perplexing.

There are three main categories of international health organizations:

9.4.1. Multilateral Organizations

Funding that is referred to as "multilateral" is provided to multiple nations by various governments and non-governmental organizations. All of the major international organizations are encompassed within the United Nations. The WHO is widely recognized as the foremost global health organization. This organization is referred to as a "Intergovernmental agency related to the United Nations" in official terminology. The WHO and other intergovernmental organizations operate independently and collaborate with the UN and each other through the coordinating machinery of the Economic and Social Council. The primary objective of the organization, as stated in its 1948 constitution, is to achieve the highest possible level of health for all people. One of the primary duties of the World Health Organization (WHO) is to offer countries technical assistance and oversee the coordination of global health initiatives. The organization engages in various activities such as:

- Establishing standards and guidelines
- Disseminating health information
- Promoting research
- Providing education on global health
- Analyzing epidemiological data
- Developing monitoring and assessment systems for health programs

The Pan American Health Organization has a unique role as the regional field office for WHO in the Americas, but it also carries out additional independent functions due to its establishment prior to WHO.

Another important intergovernmental agency connected to the UN that plays a crucial role in global health is the World Bank. Less developed countries have the opportunity to secure loans from the World Bank under highly advantageous conditions that are not typically available in the private sector. In the past decade, there has been a consistent increase in the financial support provided to developing nations for the enhancement of their human resources, specifically in the areas of health and education. The percentage of loans has experienced a significant increase over the years, starting from 5% in the early 1980s and reaching 15% in the last two years. Projections indicate that this upward trend will continue, with an expected 50% increase over the next three years.

Three subsidiary entities of the UN Economic and Social Council are dedicated to international health programs. A significant portion of the budget for UNICEF is dedicated to healthcare, focusing on the well-being of children around the world. UNICEF places a high priority on the well-being of the most vulnerable children worldwide. The organization directs a significant portion of its resources towards children under the age of five and the poorest nations on the planet. The US government is a significant donor to UNICEF. However, it is worth noting that per capita contributions from the US, including those from the private sector, are comparatively lower than those from the Netherlands, Canada, Switzerland, and the Scandinavian nations.

9.4.2. Bilateral Agencies

Bilateral agencies refer to governmental organizations in one nation that provide assistance to developing nations. The United States Agency for International Development (USAID) is the largest among these organizations. In the majority of developed countries, there are similar governmental organization that are comparable to others. Political and historical factors often play a significant role in determining which states receive funds from bilateral agencies and the amount of those gifts. As an example, Japan primarily provides donations to developing Asian nations, while France directs its attention towards its former colonies. USAID allocates millions of dollars every year towards long-term healthcare in developing nations through its Center for Population, Health, and Nutrition. A significant portion of this funding is directed towards "cooperating agencies" – private international health organizations that have contractual agreements with USAID.

9.4.3. Non-Governmental Organizations

Non-Governmental Organizations (NGOs) are entities that operate independently from the government and are driven by a specific cause or mission. They play a crucial role in addressing social, environmental, and humanitarian issues. These organizations rely on private funding and volunteers to carry out their work.

NGOs, also known as private voluntary organizations (PVOs), contribute a significant 20% of external health aid to developing nations. Most of these organizations are small in size, with several of them being affiliated with churches. Missionary societies have a distinct and crucial role in operating hospitals and clinics in some of the most impoverished nations on the planet. Based on the available data, it is evident that church mission hospitals in Uganda demonstrate a higher level of efficiency compared to government hospitals. The numbers speak for themselves – mission doctors are able to treat five times the number of patients as their government counterparts, while mission nurses attend to twice as many patients as government nurses. Project Hope – with an annual budget exceeding $100 million – holds the distinction of being the largest non-governmental organization in the United States that is solely committed to improving foreign health. Oxfam International is widely regarded as one of the most influential NGOs in the field of long-term international health.

9.5. Global Health Policies

Global health policy has a significant impact on the health and well-being of individuals and populations around the world. Numerous factors from around the world have a significant impact on national policies, societal norms, and individual health habits. It is important to recognize that many health determinants operate on a global level. Health policy makers face numerous challenges that cause anxiety. These challenges include the emergence of contagious diseases, the increasing prevalence of chronic illnesses, and the effectiveness of health systems in providing top-notch care (Holtz, 2013). The objective of global health policy is to provide individuals with a comprehensive understanding of the epidemiologic patterns in global health, the organizations responsible for global health governance, and the impact of globalization on national and global health policy. This knowledge is crucial in the face of significant social, political, and economic transformations that are posing rapid challenges to global health (Holtz, 2013).

Over the past 15 years, there has been a notable development in global health policy – the expansion and refinement of international public health law. In the past, public health was primarily considered a domain that fell under the jurisdiction of individual nations, leaving limited room for collaborative efforts on a global scale (Holtz, 2013).

While international public health law has made significant progress and continues to grow, it is important to note that domestic and national public health law remains the primary focus in this field at present. International public health law has gained significant importance in shaping national public health law and policy.

This is achieved through the establishment of legally binding standards of global health law that regulate the behavior of nations and influence their domestic actions. Additionally, the development of global norms further impacts the actions taken by individual states.

In recent times, the realm of international public health law has expanded to encompass various topics. These include:

- Biomedical science
- Human reproduction and cloning
- Organ transplantation and xenotransplantation
- Infectious and noncommunicable diseases
- Food and pharmaceutical regulation in international trade
- Regulation of dangerous and addictive substances such as tobacco and drugs

One interesting observation is the increasing connection between international health law and other established areas of international law. It is becoming more and more evident that environmental law and the regulation of toxic pollutants, arms control, the prohibition of weapons of mass destruction, human rights law, nuclear safety and radiation protection, and occupational health and safety are all closely intertwined with public health (Holtz, 2013).

Here are several examples of international law and public health:

- In 2006, the Convention on the Rights of Persons with Disabilities was established to address the rights of individuals with disabilities.
- In 2005, the International Health Regulations (revised) were put in place to focus on the control of communicable diseases.
- In 2003, the World Health Organization established the Framework Convention on Tobacco Control, which aims to address global tobacco control.
- In 1966, human rights became a significant topic of discussion.
- The World Economic, Social, and Cultural Rights Covenant.
- The Global Agreement on Civil and Political Rights of 1966.
- The Convention on Certain Conventional Weapons of 1980.
- The 1979 Convention on the Elimination of All Forms of Discrimination Against Women.
- The Convention of 1984 prohibits the use of torture and other cruel, inhuman, or degrading methods of punishment (Holtz, 2013).
- Convention on the Rights of the Child of 1989.

9.6. Cross-Cultural Health Promotion

The sociocultural backgrounds of both the patient and the provider have a significant impact on communication and clinical decision-making. Studies have shown that effective communication between healthcare providers and patients has a significant impact on patient satisfaction, adherence to treatment, and overall health outcomes (Haintz et al., 2015). Thus, when the patient and physician fail to acknowledge, analyze, comprehend, or communicate sociocultural disparities during the medical interaction, it leads to subpar compliance, negative health results, unequal treatment based on race/ethnicity, and dissatisfaction among patients.

There has been much debate and extensive discussion surrounding the concept of "culture," leading to the identification of certain recurring themes. Ultimately, culture can be described as a cohesive framework of learned concepts and actions that are collectively embraced by communities. Patterns encompass a wide range of elements, such as beliefs, attitudes, communication styles, values, practices, and conventions. Our understanding of the world is shaped by culture, which in turn affects our perception and evaluation of it (Haintz et al., 2015). One way to approach this is to consider it as an integral part of our individual identities, shaped by our various influences, rather than as something foreign or related to different groups (such as socioeconomic status, religion, gender, sexual orientation, occupation, disability, etc.). It is important to recognize that we are all influenced by a multitude of cultures that go beyond race and nationality.

It is also important to recognize the significant impact of sociocultural factors in the medical encounter. However, it is concerning that there is a lack of cross-cultural curriculum in undergraduate, graduate, and continuing education programs for health professions. The primary goal is to enhance the learner's understanding of how sociocultural factors influence health attitudes and behaviors. Additionally, these programs aim to equip learners with the necessary skills to comprehend and manage these factors during medical interactions. It is important to have a comprehensive understanding of illness prevalence, health outcomes, and ethnopharmacology within a specific population (Haintz et al., 2015).

The foundation of cross-cultural care lies in embracing the core values of professionalism. These values include humbleness, empathy, curiosity, respect, sensitivity, and awareness of all external effects on the patient. By embodying these values, healthcare professionals can provide effective and compassionate care to individuals from diverse cultural backgrounds. Curricula have been developed to address the importance of attitudes in cross-cultural medical interactions. These curricula focus on investigating and reconciling differing health beliefs and behaviors among healthcare professionals. The cultural sensitivity/awareness method incorporates educational exercises and procedures that promote self-reflection while respecting diverse health values, beliefs, and practices (Haintz et al., 2015). It is crucial to have a deep understanding of one's own culture, as well as being aware of any biases or preconceived notions that may lead to stereotypes.

Some examples involve:

- Engaging in open discussions about the impact of discrimination in the healthcare industry
- Exploring personal experiences of healthcare professionals who have felt marginalized

- Examining unconscious biases that may arise from stereotypes
- Evaluating our reactions to diverse patient images
- Discussing the experiences of our family members with the medical system

From a practical standpoint, altering attitudes requires a significant amount of effort, presents numerous challenges, evokes strong emotions, and is hard to evaluate. For those with a more clinical orientation, it may appear abstract as well. In order to ensure effective communication during the clinical encounter, it is crucial to possess qualities such as inquiry, empathy, respect, and humility, regardless of the patient's cultural background (Haintz et al., 2015).

9.7. Humanitarian Health Promotion

A humanitarian emergency is an incident or series of events that presents a significant threat to the health, safety, security, or overall well-being of a community or a large population. These emergencies often occur over a wide geographical area.

When an incident affects vulnerable populations who are unable to cope with the adverse consequences independently, it gives rise to a humanitarian emergency. Vulnerability is often linked to poverty and refers to the reduced capacity of individuals or communities to endure and bounce back from life-threatening hazards (Banatvala & Zwi, 2000). Impoverished communities face a higher vulnerability to both natural and man-made disasters. Impacted communities often have vulnerable groups, including young people, pregnant or nursing women, migrants, and internally displaced individuals.

Emergencies such as armed wars, starvation, natural catastrophes, and epidemics have the potential to lead to humanitarian disasters that are beyond the control or capacity of any single organization. Survivors of any disaster are in urgent need of essential resources such as food, water, shelter, and medical attention (Banatvala & Zwi, 2000).

Humanitarian crises can be categorized as:

- **Natural Disasters:** These can be categorized into different types based on their characteristics. These include:
  - Hydrological events like floods and avalanches
  - Climatological occurrences such as droughts
  - Meteorological phenomena like storms and cyclones
  - Geophysical incidents such as earthquakes, tsunamis, and volcanic eruptions
  - Biological events like epidemics and plagues
- **Man-Made Disasters:** These encompass a range of events, including industrial mishaps, rail and airplane wrecks, fires, and armed wars.

A humanitarian crisis arises from intricate emergencies that often encompass a combination of human-induced and natural factors, along with various vulnerabilities and a multitude of other circumstances (Banatvala & Zwi, 2000). Examples of the challenges we face include armed conflicts, the issue of food insecurity, and the displacement of populations. Complex emergencies are often marked by elevated levels of violence and fatalities. For instance:

- The phenomenon of population displacement

- Widespread damage to economies and civilizations
- The need for comprehensive and diverse humanitarian assistance
- The obstruction or hindrance of humanitarian aid due to military and political restrictions.
- In certain locations, aid workers face significant security threats

Understanding the classification of a humanitarian disaster can be quite complex. Regardless of the nature of the disaster, the initial focus of any humanitarian response is to address the urgent needs of affected individuals in order to save lives and alleviate suffering. The way in which these needs are addressed depends on the specific emergency at hand. One example is the heightened emphasis on safeguarding the well-being of humanitarian personnel in times of armed hostilities. Reaching the affected populations in the aftermath of floods or tsunamis can pose significant challenges, as highlighted by Banatvala and Zwi (2000).

Each humanitarian crisis presents a distinct set of circumstances that necessitates a tailored approach. Phenomena such as unplanned urbanization, poverty, underdevelopment, and climate change can contribute to the heightened complexity, frequency, and severity of humanitarian situations. Humanitarian health promotion aims to safeguard the well-being of communities facing the threat of natural disasters, armed conflict, or displacement. The provision of medical care goes beyond its basic function; it empowers individuals to navigate their health amidst challenging circumstances (Banatvala & Zwi, 2000).

9.7.1. Principles of Health Promotion in Humanitarian Contexts

- **Equity:** It is important to recognize that every individual, regardless of their circumstances, is entitled to access health information, services, and resources. This principle of equity ensures that everyone has an equal opportunity to obtain the necessary support for their well-being.
- **Empowerment:** Empowerment is a crucial aspect of promoting health as it fosters independence, resilience, and the ability to make thoughtful decisions (Banatvala & Zwi, 2000).
- **Holistic Approach:** A holistic approach considers various aspects of health, including social, mental, and physical well-being.
- **Cooperation:** Cooperation is greatly strengthened through alliances with regional associations, national and international organizations, as they significantly enhance their influence.

9.7.2. Challenges in Humanitarian Environments

- **Limitations on Resources:** One of the major challenges faced in health promotion initiatives is the limited availability of resources, including infrastructure, staff, and finance. These limitations can significantly hinder the progress and effectiveness of such initiatives.
- **Cultural Context:** Good communication requires an understanding of cultural norms and ideas.
- **Trauma and Mental Health:** When individuals go through a crisis, they often face challenges such as anxiety, despair, and trauma.

- **Displacement:** Individuals who are internally displaced, refugees, or migrants encounter particular difficulties.

9.7.3. Techniques for Promoting Health in an Effective Way

- **Health Education:** accurate information on nutrition, illness prevention, cleanliness, and reproductive health must be shared.
- **Behavior Change Communication:** This involves the distribution of culturally relevant messages aimed at encouraging individuals to make healthy lifestyle choices.
- **Community Mobilization:** This refers to the process of engaging and empowering communities to identify health priorities and devise effective solutions.
- **Advocacy:** This involves harnessing the perspectives and experiences of marginalized communities to bring about meaningful change in resource allocation and policy-making.

Emphasizing the importance of humanitarian health is crucial, as it is a fundamental requirement rather than a luxury. One way to transform a catastrophe into an opportunity is by advocating for health fairness, fostering community resilience, and empowering individuals (Banatvala & Zwi, 2000). Amidst the current turmoil, it is imperative that we, as health experts, legislators, and compassionate citizens, come together to advocate for the well-being of all (Figure 9.3).

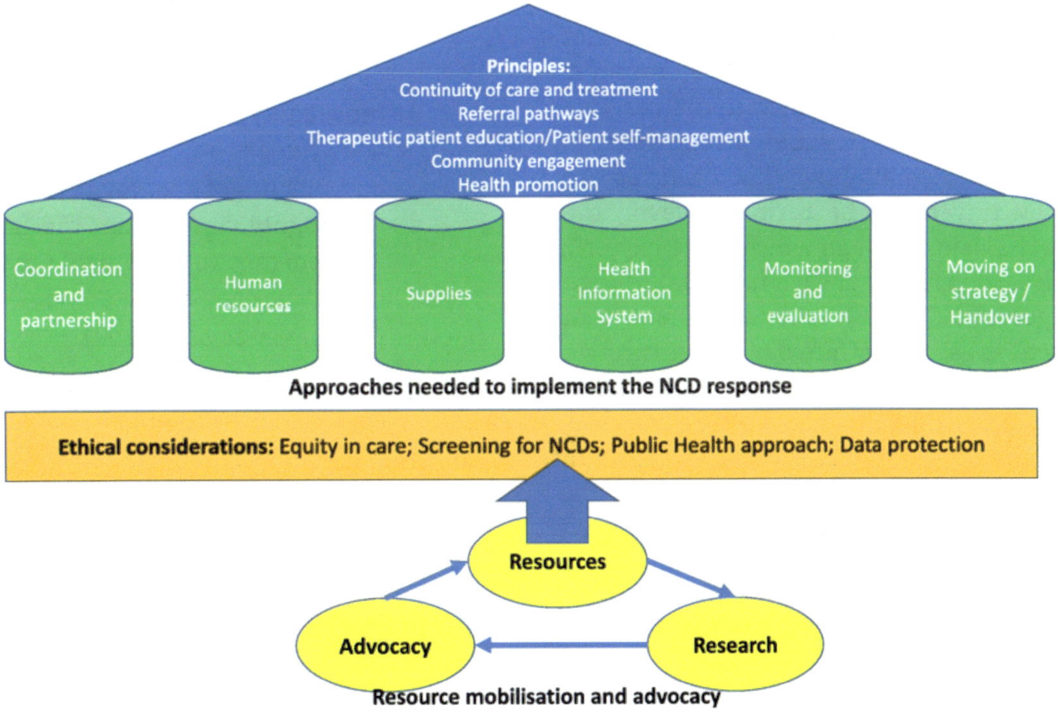

Figure 9.3. *Framework for responders to NCDs in humanitarian settings.*

Source: Bausch et al. (2021).

9.8. Preventing Infectious Diseases

Pathogens, such as bacteria, viruses, fungi, or parasites, have the ability to invade the body, spread, and interfere with normal bodily functions, ultimately leading to the development of infections. One of the leading causes of illness and death worldwide are infectious diseases. Some individuals may face greater challenges in preventing infections, particularly if they have significant injuries, are taking immune-suppressive medications, or have underlying medical conditions such as cancer or heart disease (Ellwanger et al., 2019). Nevertheless, adhering to a set of fundamental principles can greatly contribute to the prevention of infections for the majority of individuals in good health.

Having a good grasp of how infections are transmitted can be instrumental in preventing illness. It was only recently discovered that infectious diseases are caused by microscopic organisms that can be transmitted from one person to another. It is widely acknowledged in the scientific community that diseases are caused by tiny living bacteria. However, the exact mechanisms through which these bacteria cause diseases are not always fully understood (Ellwanger et al., 2019). It is understood that most bacteria gain entry into our bodies through various openings, including the mouth, nose, ears, anus, and vaginal canals. In addition, it is possible for them to enter our bodies through the skin via bites from insects or animals. One of the most effective ways to safeguard against illnesses is by implementing measures to prevent the entry of viruses into the body.

9.8.1. Good Hygiene in Preventing the Spread of Infections

Maintaining proper personal hygiene is crucial in protecting ourselves from harmful pathogens. By following these straightforward steps, individuals can effectively prevent the onset of an infection and halt its transmission to others.

- **Hands Should be Thoroughly Cleaned:** It is important to ensure that hands are thoroughly cleaned. It is important to note that washing your hands before preparing or eating meals, after using the restroom, after gardening, and after performing other unclean duties is a crucial practice. Furthermore, it is advisable to take a shower after interacting with your pet, caring for someone who is ill, or when you have blown your nose, coughed, or sneezed. It is important to ensure that your hands are thoroughly wet. Begin by creating a lather using your chosen cleanser or soap. Gently massage the lather into your wrists, palms, and the backs of your hands. It is important to thoroughly clean the spaces between your fingers, under your nails, and on your fingertips. Ensure that you thoroughly rinse under the faucet. It is important to thoroughly dry your hands and wrists, as emphasized by Ellwanger, et al., (2019).
- **Make Sure to Cover Your Cough:** It is important to remember to cover your nose and mouth with a tissue when you cough or sneeze, and promptly dispose of it. When tissue is not readily available, it is important to remember to sneeze or cough into your elbow instead of your hands.
- **Thoroughly Clean Any Cuts Before Applying a Bandage:** It is crucial for a physician to thoroughly examine any significant wounds or bites caused by humans or animals.

- Refrain from popping pimples or picking at wounds that are in the process of healing.
- Refrain from sharing your utensils, glasses, and dishes with others.
- Avoid touching items such as handkerchiefs, napkins, tissues, and other similar objects that may have been used by others.
- It is essential to implement proper food-safety practices in order to prevent any potential illnesses.

It is important to note that although most food-borne infections are generally not harmful, there is a small subset that can lead to severe illnesses such as meningitis and kidney failure (Ellwanger et al., 2019). Ensuring proper preparation and storage of food is crucial in safeguarding your family against illnesses caused by harmful bacteria. To ensure the safety of your food at home, it is important to take certain precautions. By following these steps, you can prevent the introduction of new microorganisms and eliminate any existing ones:

- It is important to ensure that all meat, poultry, fish, fruits, and vegetables are thoroughly washed under running water before preparing or serving them.
- It is important to remember to wash your hands with soap and water both before and after handling raw meat. This simple step can help prevent the spread of bacteria and keep you and your food safe.
- It is important to ensure that cooked and raw foods are kept separate from each other. It is crucial to always remember to clean your cutting boards and equipment thoroughly before using them to prepare cooked meat, especially if they were previously used to handle raw meat. This simple step helps to prevent cross-contamination and ensures the safety of your food.
- Cooking food to perfection is essential for creating a delicious and satisfying meal. It is important to ensure that the internal temperature of whole poultry reaches 180° F, while roasts and steaks should be cooked to a temperature of 145° F. Ground meats, on the other hand, should reach a temperature of 160° F. To accurately measure these temperatures, it is recommended to use a meat thermometer.
- It is important to defrost foods using either the microwave or refrigerator.

Vaccinations are crucial in order to prevent illness. In a general sense:

- It is recommended that children receive the necessary vaccines during their childhood.
- It is important for adults to ensure that their immunizations are up to date.
- Before embarking on overseas travel, it is important to have a discussion with your healthcare physician regarding the necessity of booster shots.
- Make sure to confirm that your pet has received the most up-to-date vaccines. It is important to note that ensuring the safety of your cat also has implications for the well-being of yourself and your loved ones (Ellwanger et al., 2019).

9.9. Maternal and Child Health Promotion

Maternal health encompasses the well-being of women throughout their pregnancies, deliveries, and postpartum periods. In order to optimize the health and well-being of women and their infants, it is crucial to make each stage a pleasurable experience. In 2020, a staggering 287,000 women tragically lost their lives during or after pregnancy and delivery, despite the significant advancements made in the past two decades (Organization, 2015). This number is significantly higher than expected. One must consider various factors that contribute to maternal injury and death, such as anemia, malaria, heart disease, excessive blood loss, infection, high blood pressure, botched abortion, and obstructed labor. With timely intervention from a skilled healthcare professional in a supportive environment, many maternal deaths can be prevented.

It is crucial that we maintain a strong focus on preventing maternal mortality, as it remains a pressing issue on the international agenda. Merely going through pregnancy and delivery is not enough to gauge the effectiveness of maternal health care. To enhance health and wellbeing, it is crucial to implement more strategies focused on preventing maternal injury and disability. According to studies, each conception and delivery is unique. In order to ensure that all women have equal access to compassionate and high-quality maternity care, it is crucial to tackle the inequalities that affect health outcomes, especially those related to gender and sexual and reproductive health and rights.

Participating in health promotion programs that focus on the health and wellbeing of pregnant women can greatly enhance early childhood outcomes. The Life Course Framework is a valuable tool in understanding the intricate connections between maternal experiences and the health outcomes of their unborn children. By examining the experiences and exposures of pregnant women, we can gain insights into the potential impacts on early childhood health. Based on this concept, an individual's health gradually improves as they integrate healthy environmental, behavioral, mental, and physical activities into their daily routine. On the other hand, it is worth noting that an individual's health tends to deteriorate as they continue to partake in detrimental or negative behaviors. Optimal birth outcomes and optimal childhood health are observed in the children of pregnant women who exhibit positive physical, mental, environmental, and behavioral health throughout their lives. Research has shown that the risk factors children are exposed to during the critical 1,000-day period from conception to their second birthday play a significant role in the development of childhood obesity and related illnesses (Organization, 2015).

Maintaining a healthy weight is a proactive measure that women of reproductive age can adopt to enhance the well-being of their children. According to a study conducted in 2014, it was found that in the most rural counties in the United States, more than 40% of women over the age of 18 reported themselves as being obese (Organization, 2015). Maternal obesity is associated with an increased risk of preterm birth, gestational diabetes, preeclampsia, having a large baby, and stillbirth. In addition, it is worth noting that maternal obesity is a significant factor when it comes to determining childhood obesity. It is highly recommended that women of childbearing age receive preconception care (a form of preventive treatment) prior to getting pregnant. The organization provides comprehensive guidance and instruction on various aspects of health, including behavioral, mental, emotional, and physical well-being. Its aim is to promote the best possible outcomes for both mother and child (Organization, 2015).

During the early stages of pregnancy, regular prenatal visits can provide valuable benefits for expectant mothers. Prenatal care includes educating individuals on healthy habits to adopt during pregnancy and creating an ideal environment for the development of the fetus (Organization, 2015). During these visits, the health of both the mother and baby is assessed to ensure a positive delivery experience. Aside from emphasizing the importance of doctor visits and prenatal care, programs may choose to prioritize various other factors that impact children's health. These may include reducing or eliminating exposure to dangerous substances, such as lead, addressing drug abuse and mental health issues during and after pregnancy, and offering a variety of community resources and services to assist women and families with their health and social needs.

9.10. Global Health Governance (GHG)

Governance is the term used to describe the different ways in which people come together to achieve common goals. In order for collective action to take place, it is crucial to adhere to established institutions, norms, and rules. These include resource mobilization and allocation, decision-making processes, authority distribution, communication channels, and membership in cooperative relationships (Kumar & Preetha, 2012). Health governance encompasses a set of established guidelines, customs, and establishments that collaborate to protect and promote health.

It is crucial to note that governance encompasses the involvement of different social actors, such as the corporate sector and civil society organizations (CSOs), alongside the government's significant role. In addition, governance covers a broad spectrum of official methods, including laws, treaties, and codes of practice, as well as informal methods like norms and customs. Formal agreements with regulatory authorities carry legal weight and can be backed by punitive measures such as fines or incarceration. Informal systems often incorporate various forms of criticism, including public opinion, self-regulation, and voluntary compliance (Kumar & Preetha, 2012).

9.10.1. Differences Between Global Health Governance (GHG) and International Health Governance (IHG)

Global Health Governance (GHG) and international health governance (IHG) have distinct differences that set them apart from each other.

First, IHG involves the crucial aspect of cross-border collaboration between governments. These governments share a common goal, which is the welfare and wellbeing of their respective citizens. IHG encompasses various aspects such as the surveillance, reporting, and monitoring of infectious diseases, the regulation of trade in health services, and the protection of patented medications under the Agreement on Trade-Related Intellectual Property Rights (TRIPS). Globalization has led to an increase in the complexity of health factors and outcomes, making it challenging to confine them within a single territorial boundary, such as a country. In some cases, these factors have even become detached from physical location (Kumar & Preetha, 2012). Furthermore, when it comes to power and enforcement, it is important to note that governments are the central focus of IHG processes. Two notable examples include the Framework Convention on Tobacco Control (FCTC) and the International Health Regulations (IHR).

On the other hand, GHG covers a wide range of official and informal governance structures, including both governmental and non-governmental entities. These include codes of conduct that are optional, quality assurance standards, accreditation procedures, and customer tracking and reporting. These mechanisms vary significantly in terms of their scope, aim, jurisdiction, and auxiliary resources (Kumar & Preetha, 2012). Additionally, GHG takes into consideration various factors that influence health, such as trade, finance, and the environment, at different levels of governance. In contrast, IHG primarily concentrates on the health sector (Kumar & Preetha, 2012).

In order to effectively address health determinants, status, and outcomes, it is crucial to recognize that actions taken solely at the national level will not be enough. In today's interconnected world, where health hazards and opportunities are increasingly integrated on a global scale, a broader approach is required. It is imperative to reassess the laws and organizations governing health policy and practice in response to the growing movement of people, ideas, goods, and services across borders. Given the impact of globalization on health, it becomes imperative to reevaluate traditional approaches to health promotion. It is crucial to recognize the impact of globalization on individuals' capacity to enhance and assert control over their health (Kumar & Preetha, 2012).

Globalization refers to the process of enhancing the exchange of people, trade, finance, knowledge, and ideas across borders. For instance: It might be necessary to pay more attention to the changing patterns of population movement within and between nations, like migration, tourism, displaced people, and migrant labor, in order to promote sexual health.

It may be imperative to implement measures to counteract the marketing efforts of multinational corporations promoting global brands, with the aim of encouraging healthier eating habits. Promoting tobacco control requires addressing the issue of illegal cigarettes and multinational tobacco corporations' focus on developing markets in low- and middle-income countries. The impact of large-scale agriculture production on urbanization and land availability should be carefully considered when planning for healthy living environments.

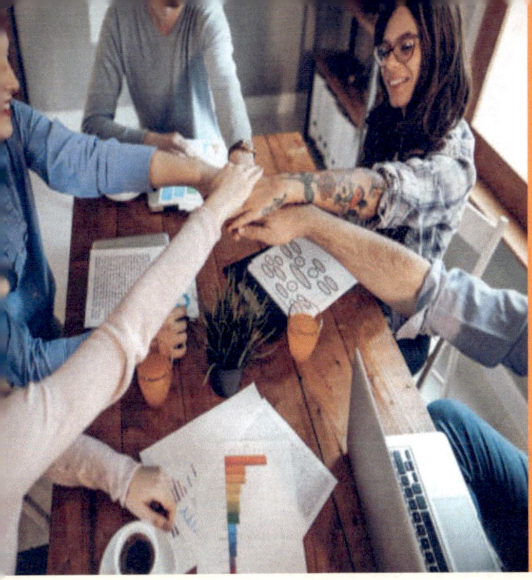

Chapter 10

ETHICS IN HEALTH PROMOTION

Contents

Ethics in health promotion guides the interconnection between compassion, public health, and social responsibility. It strongly prioritizes empowerment, equity, and community engagement. Within humanitarian contexts, ethical challenges arise due to factors such as trauma, cultural norms, and resource constraints. The ethical imperative is to balance the societal needs with the welfare of the individual. Health promotion has the potential to transform disasters into chances for a superior and healthier global environment by embracing ethical principles outlined below.

- **Beneficence:** This is the principle that requires healthcare professionals to act in the best interest of their patients. It includes protecting and defending the patient's rights, avoiding harm, removing harmful conditions, assisting those with disabilities, and rescuing people in danger. Beneficence goes beyond nonmaleficence, which simply requires not causing harm. It is important for healthcare professionals to promote the welfare of their patients and benefit them in addition to preventing harm.

- **Nonmaleficence:** According to this principle, healthcare professionals have an ethical duty to not harm their patients. This includes not causing pain or suffering, not rendering someone helpless, not inciting hatred, and not denying another person their basic human rights. Healthcare professionals use the principle of nonmaleficence in practice by weighing the benefits and risks of interventions and treatments, avoiding those that are unduly taxing, and selecting the best course of action for the patient. This principle is particularly relevant in difficult decisions regarding life-sustaining therapy, nutrition and hydration, and pain management.
- **Autonomy:** According to this principle, every adult human with a sound mind has the right to make decisions about their own body. Healthcare professionals are obligated to provide patients with the necessary information and treatment options to exercise their right to self-determination. However, individuals who are unable to make decisions for themselves, such as young children or those with developmental, mental, or physical disorders, are not covered by the principle of autonomy. There is also a debate about the concept of autonomy, with some suggesting a more expansive idea of relational autonomy that takes into account social interactions and factors such as gender, race, and culture.
- **Justice:** This principle calls for fair, equitable, and suitable treatment of individuals. In the context of clinical ethics, distributive justice is the most relevant type of justice. It refers to the justifiable principles that govern the allocation of healthcare resources. Different principles of distributive justice include equal share, need-based, effort-based, contribution-based, merit-based, and free-market trades. These principles are often combined and applied in different ways to ensure fair distribution of healthcare resources.
- Overall, ethics in health promotion is crucial for balancing the needs of society with the welfare of the individual. It requires healthcare professionals to act in the best interest of their patients, avoid causing harm, respect the patient's autonomy, and ensure fair distribution of resources. By embracing ethical ideals, health promotion can turn catastrophes into opportunities for a better and healthier world.

10.1. Ethical Issues in Health Promotion

The ethical issues in health promotion can be categorized into two main concerns: efficacy-based and autonomy-based. Efficacy-based concerns question the effectiveness and cost-effectiveness of health promotion strategies. Autonomy-based focus on whether health promotion efforts try to control social values and lifestyles, and to what extent they impede on individuals' free will (Tones & Tilford, 2001).

Determining the appropriate techniques to enhance health is a contentious ethical issue in health promotion. The term "appropriate" can be interpreted as the most economically efficient way to achieve goals or the morally just way to do so. The cost and efficacy of health promotion strategies are significant issues, as there is a need to define what constitutes an effective strategy and how to evaluate health promotion tactics.

Health promotion interventions can range from disseminating knowledge through instruction to manipulating or forcing preferences. Behavior change strategies often target specific lifestyle objectives (such as quitting smoking or increasing physical activity) and employ various tactics to influence the target population. However, these tactics raise concerns about their impact on people's lifestyles. For example, stigmatizing and discriminating against individuals in polygamous relationships based on the belief that such relationships are dangerous and unethical may have unintended consequences (Tones & Tilford, 2001). It is also important to consider whether monogamy should be valued above other values, even if it has positive social effects. Additionally, there may be moral conflicts between medical truths, such as the transmission of HIV through unprotected intercourse, and underlying moral judgments about having multiple sexual partners.

Health promotion also raises questions about the role of government intervention in shaping or influencing people's decisions. Liberal societies generally believe that decisions about lifestyle and behavior should be left up to individuals, but there is recognition that government intervention may be justified in certain cases. The moral implications of government policies for health promotion or attempts to alter behavior need to be considered.

Some health promotion initiatives may fail to respect an individual's right to autonomy, or the freedom to make choices about their own lives. Persuasion, particularly when used by authoritative professionals, can be problematic if it disregards the wishes of individuals or groups and applies pressure to follow the advice given. Manipulation and deception are also ethical concerns in health promotion. Manipulation involves purposefully swaying people's views by non-persuasively changing their understanding of a situation, while deception involves lying, hiding facts, or creating false impressions (Tones & Tilford, 2001).

10.2. Informed Consent

Informed consent is the procedure by which a healthcare practitioner provides a patient with comprehensive information regarding the benefits, drawbacks, and alternative choices for a specific medical treatment or intervention. Prior to making a decision regarding the operation or intervention, it is imperative that the patient possesses the necessary competence to do so of their own free will. Healthcare personnel have a legal and moral obligation in most systems to ensure that patients provide informed consent (Buchanan, 2000). This concept can be applied to a broader range of activities beyond healthcare interventions, including research and the disclosure of an individual's medical information. Obtaining informed consent is not always required. If an individual is considered unable to provide informed consent, it is generally allowed for another person to provide consent on their behalf. Instances of such individuals encompass conservators responsible for individuals with mental illness and parents or legal guardians of minors (although in certain situations, the minor may be obligated to provide informed assent). In specific circumstances, the theory of informed consent permits treatment as an alternative, such as when an unconscious individual is nearing death and immediate intervention is not possible. Insufficient information provided to individuals can lead to significant ethical dilemmas, as they are unable to make well-informed decisions (Buchanan, 2000). If these issues occur or are anticipated to occur in a clinical trial, they may be evaluated by an institutional review board or an ethical committee. Assessing informed consent can be difficult because the act of expressing consent or having knowledge of its consequences does not necessarily indicate that complete adult consent was given or that all relevant information was fully understood. Consent can be implied through subtle cues in everyday communication, rather than explicitly discussed in written or spoken form. A patient can indicate their consent when a doctor proposes to measure their blood pressure, for instance, by extending their arm to facilitate the placement of a blood pressure cuff. Despite the subject's assertion of understanding and desire for a different outcome, there exist circumstances in which consent lacks legal enforceability (Buchanan, 2000). While there is presently no flawless tool, there are systematic methods for evaluating the capacity to provide informed consent.

Consequently, there is consistently a point at which informed consent must be assumed or inferred based on knowledge, observation, or legal precedent. This is especially applicable in cases of sexual or relationship difficulties. Irrespective of authentic authorization, explicit consent through a signature, which is usually legally relied upon, is the norm in medical or formal situations. Some operations, such as a patient signing a "do not resuscitate" order before their illness begins, are indeed true (Buchanan, 2000).

Below are a few examples of each of the aforementioned:

1. An individual may choose to relinquish something willingly due to fear, societal expectations, or a psychological inhibition in expressing their true emotions. The person making the request may be genuinely unaware of this and is relying on approval. Verbal consent is not given here.
2. An individual may seem to comprehend the consequences of an action when granting permission, but in truth, they may not fully grasp the possible outcomes. Consequently, they may later dispute the validity of their consent. Despite the presence of the necessary understanding, ignorance hinders the ability to give informed consent.
3. Following the completion of a formal release document for a medical procedure, the patient harbors doubts regarding the authenticity of their consent. In legal terms, the release is usually considered definitive or persuasive, allowing the doctor to legally depend on it for consent, unless he can provide evidence of a true mistake. In formal situations, a written consent usually holds more legal weight than a later refusal of informed consent, unless it was obtained through deceit (Buchanan, 2000).

10.3. Confidentiality and Privacy

These are essential aspects of maintaining trust and respecting an individual's rights in various professional relationships, including healthcare. Privacy refers to the right to be free from interference and control over personal information, while confidentiality is the obligation to preserve privileged information and communicate entrusted information sensibly (Terry & Francis, 2007). In healthcare, healthcare professionals have a responsibility to keep private and medical information confidential, unless the patient gives permission to disclose it.

The Health Insurance Portability and Accountability Act of 1996 (HIPAA) was established to protect patient data in medical records and set guidelines for the transmission and sharing of electronic data (Terry & Francis, 2007). HIPAA requires healthcare professionals to obtain a patient's permission before sharing private information with third parties. Patients should receive a written notice of privacy practices, which outlines their rights and the safeguards in place to protect their personal and medical information. HIPAA also regulates marketing tactics to prevent the sale and distribution of patient data without consent.

Privacy and confidentiality are not absolute concepts and can vary depending on the situation. The reasonable expectation of privacy may decrease if personal information is shared in a public setting. However, discussing medical information in a private office can help preserve privacy (Terry & Francis, 2007).

While healthcare professionals generally require patient consent before disclosing information, there are rare situations where confidentiality obligations may be superseded by concerns for justice and the greater good. For example, a court order may require a doctor to provide a patient's information without their agreement. Additionally, if a doctor believes a patient poses a clear danger to others, they may have a "duty to warn" the appropriate authorities (Terry & Francis, 2007).

It is important to recognize the privacy and anonymity needs of elderly patients. Even if family, friends, or healthcare staff may think privacy is unimportant for older patients, they may still value their privacy. Regardless of age, patients should expect that any information they share with a healthcare team will be kept confidential. Upholding confidentiality can give older patients a sense of autonomy and control over their lives, even while in the hospital. Healthcare personnel should not assume that an older patient wants family and friends present in the hospital room without their explicit consent (Terry & Francis, 2007).

10.4. Conflicts of Interest in Health Promotion

Conflicts of interest (COI) in health promotion occur when individuals or organizations are biased in their judgment, decisions, and actions due to personal interests, financial considerations, or favoritism. COI can be categorized as financial or nonfinancial (Motola, Devine, et al., 2013). Financial COI includes monetary interests such as ownership of shares or business transactions, while nonfinancial COI refers to biases stemming from friendships, family ties, or personal factors. Common examples of COI include nepotism, self-dealing, and excessive compensation.

In the healthcare industry, conflicts of interest can arise between doctors, administrators, and patients. These conflicts can have negative effects on roles, relationships, clinical evidence, public opinion, treatment decisions, research integrity, and the independence of laboratories. For example, medical staff may receive gifts or money from pharmaceutical companies or research centers in exchange for their participation. They may also hold shares in these businesses or receive travel expenses to attend meetings or congresses. Additionally, medical professionals may work with organizations or companies outside of their primary workplace, which can lead to conflicts of interest (Motola, Devine et al., 2013). These relationships can subtly influence a doctor's diagnosis, judgment, decision-making, and the education they provide to trainees and students. For instance, a doctor who owns stock in a pharmaceutical company may promote or suggest a specific medication, even if there are comparable alternatives available. They may also instruct medical students on the use of specific drugs. Furthermore, physicians who own testing facilities or treatment centers may recommend their patients to these facilities, potentially benefiting financially from diagnostic or treatment procedures. It is important to recognize and address conflicts of interest in health promotion to ensure unbiased decision-making and the best interests of patients. Strategies to manage COI include transparency, disclosure, and the establishment of policies and guidelines. Transparency involves openly acknowledging and discussing potential conflicts of interest. Disclosure requires individuals to disclose their financial and nonfinancial interests to relevant parties. Policies and guidelines can help regulate and manage conflicts of interest, ensuring that decisions are made in the best interest of patients and the public (Motola, Devine et al., 2013).

10.5. Equity and Social Justice

Equity and social justice are fundamental principles in promoting health and addressing health disparities. Social justice aims to eliminate structural injustices and ensure equal rights, opportunities, and respect for all individuals. Health equity goes beyond healthcare access and focuses on addressing the underlying causes of health disparities such as racism, poverty, and unfair resource allocation. It is based on the moral principles of human rights and equitable distribution of resources and opportunities (Ruger, 2004). There is a need for health equity because social factors like income, education, housing, and employment significantly influence health outcomes. Marginalized communities are particularly affected by these structural factors, leading to health disparities based on socioeconomic class, gender, race, and ethnicity. These disparities are unjust and avoidable, and addressing them is essential for achieving social justice (Ruger, 2004). The moral basis for health equity lies in recognizing health as a basic human right. Every individual should have access to the best possible level of health, regardless of their background or circumstances. Achieving equity requires the fair distribution of resources, opportunities, and rewards, challenging privilege, and promoting inclusivity. Health equity is not only about addressing health disparities but also about addressing the underlying social determinants of health (Ruger, 2004).

However, there are obstacles to encouraging health equity.

- Power dynamics play a significant role, as dismantling power structures is necessary to address injustices.
- There may be opposition to advocacy for oppressed communities, making it challenging to achieve equity.
- Cultural competence is also crucial in health promotion, as it requires understanding different worldviews and beliefs.
- Intersectionality, which acknowledges intersecting identities such as race, gender, and disability, is essential for designing customized interventions.

To promote health equity, it is important to involve impacted communities in decision-making through community engagement.

Their insights and experiences can guide effective initiatives. Policy advocacy is also crucial, supporting legislation that prohibits discrimination, provides access to affordable housing, and advances equity in healthcare. Health literacy, the ability to navigate complex health systems, is another important strategy for promoting equity (Ruger, 2004). Promoting health equity can have a change-releasing effect. By addressing social determinants, health promotion can help reduce disparities and close health inequities. Fair interventions that provide marginalized groups with a platform and foster resilience can encourage positive change. Ultimately, building just systems and creating a more equitable society as a whole benefit from health equity (Ruger, 2004). In the context of race, racism is a social construct that establishes a value system centered on Whiteness. Black, Indigenous, and People of Color (BIPOC) populations, as well as other marginalized groups, are disproportionately affected by the social determinants of health – including racism, income inequality, and gender discrimination. Structural racism, perpetuated by laws, institutions, policies, and historical injustices, contributes to the disparities experienced by these communities. For example, Indigenous peoples in Canada face poverty, homelessness, denial of rights, and worse health outcomes due to structural racism and colonialism (Ruger, 2004).

10.6. Areas of Responsibility for Health Education Specialists

The Eight Areas of Responsibility outlined by Koelen and Ban (2023) provide a comprehensive framework for the professional responsibilities of health education specialists. These areas include:

i. Determining needs and capabilities
ii. Scheduling
iii. Execution
iv. Assessment and investigation
v. Promotion
vi. Interaction
vii. Administration and guidance
viii. Morality and expertise

In Area I, health education specialists are responsible for conducting a needs assessment to identify program priorities and select effective solutions. This involves gathering and examining primary and secondary data, as well as evaluating available resources (Koelen & Ban, 2023).

Area II focuses on scheduling, which involves evaluating the health requirements, issues, and resources of the prioritized population. This is done in collaboration with partners and stakeholders to develop the mission, goals, objectives, and strategies of the program. Securing funding, organizing program delivery, and considering assessment strategies are also important tasks in this area.

Execution, covered in Area III, involves organizing staff and volunteer training, implementing program delivery strategies, tracking progress, and assessing program success. Health education specialists must consider the priority population's awareness of the health issue and address participation incentives and constraints. Collaboration with stakeholders is crucial for a well-coordinated and effective program implementation.

Area IV focuses on assessment and investigation, which is essential for determining whether program objectives have been met and for evaluating program effectiveness. Health education specialists are responsible for conducting assessments and utilizing research skills to ensure that programs are data-driven and evidence-based (Koelen & Ban, 2023).

Promotion, the focus of Area V, involves advocating for health-improving policies, regulations, and practices. Health education specialists play a crucial role in promoting changes in policy, resource allocation, and health equity. They engage the community in advocacy activities and inform prospective employers about the benefits of employing qualified and certified health education professionals. In Area VI, interaction, health education specialists interact with various individuals, including colleagues, employers, students, customers, and health professionals. Effective communication skills are essential for building and maintaining health education programs. Specialists use their expertise to create, modify, distribute, and evaluate communication messages through different platforms (Koelen & Ban, 2023).

Area VII focuses on administration and guidance, which requires effective leadership and management skills. Health education specialists recruit and involve partners and stakeholders, evaluate their capacity, and manage resources. They develop a long-term vision, collaborate to create and implement strategic plans, and oversee the management of people, money, and material resources.

Finally, in Area VIII, health education specialists are expected to maintain professionalism and ethical behavior throughout the entire process. This includes needs analysis, program development, execution, management, assessment, communication, and research. Adhering to established guidelines, engaging in ongoing education, and participating in professional societies are important aspects of professionalism in the field (Koelen & Ban, 2023).

10.7. Cultural Competence in Health Promotion

Cultural competence in health promotion is essential for providing efficient and high-quality care to patients from diverse cultural backgrounds. It involves tailoring healthcare to individual cultural and language variations, as well as being aware of the potential influence of cultural differences on healthcare provision (Kirmayer, 2012). Factors such as race, socioeconomic status, and health literacy can affect how patients perceive their ailments, seek medical attention, and adhere to treatment plans. Cultural competence in healthcare is not limited to racial and ethnic groups but also includes LGBTQIA+ individuals, persons with disabilities, and people from various socioeconomic backgrounds (Kirmayer, 2012).

One of the reasons cultural competence is important in healthcare is because differences between patients and healthcare professionals can impact communication and treatment decisions. Misunderstandings can occur when healthcare professionals misinterpret a patient's behavior or fail to acknowledge their cultural differences. Developing intercultural communication skills is crucial for providing equitable healthcare. Assembling teams of healthcare workers who represent the diversity of patient populations can also enhance cross-cultural communication and responsiveness to cultural needs (Kirmayer, 2012).

Language accessibility is another important aspect of cultural competence in healthcare. Language barriers can hinder communication between patients and doctors, leading to inaccurate descriptions of symptoms or explanations of diagnoses. Language limitations can also lead to inappropriate and dangerous situations.

Cultural diversity in healthcare matters because it influences the patient's trust in their healthcare providers. Trust is crucial for improving health equity, and cultural diversity in healthcare acknowledges and represents a wide range of communities. Studies have shown that patients rate the quality of care higher when their physicians share their racial and ethnic background, highlighting the importance of cultural diversity in the medical field (Kirmayer, 2012).

According to Kirmaye (2012), to promote cultural competence in healthcare, it is important to provide health workers with appropriate training on cultural competency and cross-cultural challenges. Policies that reduce administrative and linguistic barriers to patient care should also be developed. By implementing these strategies, healthcare organizations and practitioners can eliminate racial and ethnic health disparities, enhance health outcomes, and improve the quality of care provided to patients (Kirmayer, 2012).

10.8. Advocacy and Empowerment

These are crucial strategies in health promotion to address societal inequities and improve health outcomes. Advocacy involves bringing about change at both systemic and individual levels by giving voice to marginalized groups and opposing discriminatory laws and procedures. On the other hand, empowerment is the foundation of health promotion, giving individuals and communities the power to determine their own health outcomes through agency, autonomy, and resilience (Cyril et al., 2016).

There are two predominant models in health promotion: medical and social. The medical model focuses on preventing or treating clinically defined illnesses and relies on factual data to promote healthy behaviors. It often takes a therapeutic and individualistic approach. In contrast, the social health promotion model aims to address societal inequities and improve the lives of those who are less privileged. It focuses on the structural causes of health disparities (Cyril et al., 2016).

To achieve health equity, which involves justice and the removal of barriers, empowerment and advocacy are essential. Lomas' critique highlights the need for public health to consider both social system reform and individualist ethics. Advocacy fills this gap by promoting ethical behavior and campaigning for change (Cyril et al., 2016).

There are various techniques for advocacy and empowerment in health promotion.

- **Community Engagement:** This involves involving impacted communities in decision-making processes to ensure their voices are heard.
- **Policy Advocacy:** This aims to push for laws and policies that advance justice and equity.
- **Health Literacy:** This is another important aspect, equipping individuals with information and skills to make informed choices about their health.

10.9. Ethical Decision Making in Health Promotion

Ethical decision-making is crucial in healthcare organizations when resolving conflicts or uncertainties involving conflicting values. Healthcare executives must consider ethical principles such as fairness, autonomy, beneficence, and nonmaleficence, in addition to professional and organizational ethical standards and rules. Various factors, including equitable access and affordability, quality, patient safety, allocation of resources, and advancements in medical treatment, have contributed to the growing concern over ethical issues in healthcare organizations (Koelen & Ban, 2023). To effectively address these moral conundrums, healthcare executives should not make decisions on their own but instead follow a systematic decision-making process that considers different perspectives (Koelen & Ban, 2023). This process helps leaders, employees, and stakeholders navigate morally difficult circumstances. Healthcare leaders have a responsibility to uphold the organization's vision and values, promote an ethical culture, establish standards and accountability, and serve as examples of ethical behavior. They also have an obligation to address clinical ethical challenges at larger organizational, community, and societal levels through a systematic approach (Koelen & Ban, 2023).

According to Koelen and Ban (2023), to fulfill these responsibilities, healthcare executives should:

1. Establish an ethical culture based on the organization's vision and values by applying a systematic ethics decision-making process. This promotes moral clinical and administrative practices, policies, and decision-making.
2. Declare the organization's commitment to aligning its purpose or value declarations with ethics.
3. Set an example of moral decision-making and emphasize the importance of ethics by adhering to professional conduct standards.
4. Provide educational programs on the organization's ethical standards of practice and the global concerns that require ethical decision-making in healthcare. This includes educating individuals on making ethical decisions with patients and their families while considering cultural differences and avoiding implicit bias. Healthcare leaders can also encourage learning opportunities that foster informed and considerate debates on ethical concerns.
5. Ensure that organizational resources for handling ethical issues are easily accessible and staffed by qualified individuals. Establishing a dedicated committee to handle organizational ethics issues may be necessary, and committee members should come from diverse backgrounds to accurately represent the groups affected by recommendations or policy directives. Continuous ethical training should also be provided to ethics resources.
6. Consult resources and subject matter experts in ethics when there is doubt about an ethical issue. Leaders dealing with clinical issues should consider engaging with a qualified ethicist. Encouraging others to use organizational resources to address moral dilemmas is also important.
7. Continuously assess and improve organizational procedures for handling moral dilemmas.
8. Encourage decision-making that promotes the proper distribution of power regarding individuals, organizations, and society. Decision-making procedures should recognize and protect against privilege and ensure the fair consideration of marginalized or vulnerable individuals.

By following these guidelines, healthcare executives can effectively navigate ethical challenges and promote ethical behavior within their organizations (Koelen & Ban, 2023).

BIBLIOGRAPHY

1. Agnikula, K., Kshatriya, B. S., & Balls-Berry, J. J. (2021). Social and behavioral determinants of health in the era of artificial intelligence with electronic health records: A scoping review. *Health Data Science, 2021*(1), 1–9.
2. Ahlsvvede, R. (1971). Multi-way communication channels. In *Proc. 2nd Int. Symp. Inf. Theory*.
3. Ahmad, N. S., Musa, R., & Harun, M. H. M. (2016). The impact of social media content marketing (SMCM) towards brand health. *Procedia Economics and Finance, 37*, 331–336.
4. Ahn, S., Basu, R., Smith, M. L., Jiang, L., Lorig, K., Whitelaw, N., & Ory, M. G. (2013). The impact of chronic disease self-management programs: Healthcare savings through a community-based intervention. *BMC Public Health, 13*(1), 1–6.
5. Ajzen, I. (1991). The theory of planned behavior. *Organizational Behavior and Human Decision Processes, 50*(2), 179–211.
6. Andrus, M. R., & Roth, M. T. (2002). Health literacy: A review. *Pharmacotherapy: The Journal of Human Pharmacology and Drug Therapy, 22*(3), 282 302.
7. Baeten, R., Spasova, S., Vanhercke, B., & Coster, S. (2018). Inequalities in access to healthcare. A study of national policies. *European Social Policy Network (ESPN)*. Brussels: European Commission.
8. Baker, P., Dworkin, S. L., Tong, S., Banks, I., Shand, T., & Yamey, G. (2014). The men's health gap: Men must be included in the global health equity agenda. *Bulletin of the World Health Organization, 92*, 618–620.
9. Banatvala, N., & Zwi, A. B. (2000). Public health and humanitarian interventions: Developing the evidence base. *BMJ, 321*(7253), 101–105.
10. Beauchamp, T. L., & Childress, J. F. (2001). *Principles of Biomedical Ethics*. Oxford University Press.
11. Bergeron, K., Abdi, S., DeCorby, K., Mensah, G., Rempel, B., & Manson, H. (2017). Theories, models and frameworks used in capacity building interventions relevant to public health: A systematic review. *BMC Public Health, 17*(1), 1–12.
12. Bramantoro, T., Santoso, C. M. A., Hariyani, N., Setyowati, D., Zulfiana, A. A., Nor, N. A. M., & Irmalia, W. R. (2021). Effectiveness of the school-based oral health promotion programmes from preschool to high school: A systematic review. *PLOS ONE, 16*(8), e0256007.

13. Braveman, P. (2006). Health disparities and health equity: Concepts and measurement. *Annual Review of Public Health, 27*, 167–194.
14. Buchanan, D. R. (2000). *An ethic for Health Promotion: Rethinking the Sources of Human Well-Being*. Oxford University Press.
15. Bunnell, R., O'Neil, D., Soler, R., Payne, R., Giles, W. H., Collins, J., & Communities Putting Prevention to Work Program Group. (2012). Fifty communities putting prevention to work: Accelerating chronic disease prevention through policy, systems, and environmental change. *Journal of Community Health, 37*(5), 1081–1090.
16. Bussey, K., & Bandura, A. (1999). Social cognitive theory of gender development and differentiation. *Psychological Review, 106*(4), 676.
17. Chiu, L. (2009). Culturally competent health promotion: The potential of participatory video for empowering migrant and minority ethnic communities. *International Journal of Migration, Health and Social Care, 5*(1), 5–14.
18. Cislaghi, B., Denny, E. K., Cissé, M., Gueye, P., Shrestha, B., Shrestha, P. N., & Clark, C. J. (2019). Changing social norms: The importance of "organized diffusion" for scaling up community health promotion and women empowerment interventions. *Prevention Science, 20*, 936–946.
19. Cyril, S., Smith, B. J., Possamai-Inesedy, A., & Renzaho, A. M. N. (2016). Systematic review of empowerment measures in health promotion. *Health Promotion International, 31*(4), 809–826.
20. D'Andreamatteo, A., Ianni, L., Lega, F., & Sargiacomo, M. (2015). Lean in healthcare: A comprehensive review. *Health Policy, 119*(9), 1197–1209.
21. Dantas, J., Lumbus, A., & Gower, S. (2018). Empowerment and health promotion of refugee women. Faculty of Health Sciences, Curtin University.
22. Deci, E. L., & Ryan, R. M. (2012). Self-determination theory. In P. A. M. Van Lange, A. W. Kruglanski, & E. T. Higgins (Eds.), *Handbook of Theories of Social Psychology* (Vol. 1, pp. 416–436). Sage Publications.
23. Dickerson, D., Baldwin, J. A., Belcourt, A., Belone, L., Gittelsohn, J., Keawe'aimoku Kaholokula, J., & Wallerstein, N. (2020). Encompassing cultural contexts within scientific research methodologies in the development of health promotion interventions. *Prevention Science, 21*, 33–42.
24. Dimitrov, D. V. (2016). Medical internet of things and big data in healthcare. *Healthcare Informatics Research, 22*(3), 156.
25. Dodgson, R., Lee, K., & Drager, N. (2017). Global health governance, a conceptual review. In R. Beaglehole & R. Bonita (Eds.), *Global Health* (pp. 439–461). Oxford University Press.
26. Dressler, W. W., & Oths, K. S. (1997). Cultural determinants of health behavior. In D. S. Gochman (Ed.), *Handbook of Health Behavior Research I: Personal and Social Determinants* (pp. 359–378). Springer.
27. Ellwanger, J. H., de Lima Kaminski, V., & Chies, J. A. B. (2019). Emerging infectious disease prevention: Where should we invest our resources and efforts? *Journal of Infection and Public Health, 12*(3), 313–316.
28. Farrer, L., Marinetti, C., Cavaco, Y. K., & Costongs, C. (2015). Advocacy for health equity: A synthesis review. *The Milbank Quarterly, 93*(2), 392–437.

29. Fawzy, S., Osman, A. I., Yang, T., Doran, J., & Rooney, D. W. (2020). Strategies for mitigation of climate change: A review. *Environmental Chemistry Letters, 18*, 2069–2094.

30. Fragala, M. S., Shiffman, D., & Birse, C. E. (2019). Population health screenings for the prevention of chronic disease progression. *American Journal of Managed Care, 25*(11), 548–553.

31. Francis, T. B. (2016). Assessing the role of faith-based organizations in health promotion. The University of Tennessee Health Science Center.

32. Gaziano, T. A., Galea, G., & Reddy, K. S. (2007). Scaling up interventions for chronic disease prevention: The evidence. *The Lancet, 370*(9603), 1939–1946.

33. Goeppinger, J. (1993). Health promotion for rural populations: Partnership interventions. *Family & Community Health, 16*(1), 1–10.

34. Golding, P., & Murdock, G. (1978). Theories of communication and theories of society. *Communication Research, 5*(3), 339–356.

35. Goodman, N. M. (1971). *International Health Organizations and Their Work* (2nd ed.). Churchill Livingstone.

36. Gorgenyi-Hegyes, E., Nathan, R. J., & Fekete-Farkas, M. (2021). Workplace health promotion, employee wellbeing and loyalty during COVID-19 Pandemic—Large scale empirical evidence from Hungary. *Economies, 9*(2), 55.

37. Grossman, M. (2017). *Determinants of Health: An Economic Perspective.* Columbia University Press.

38. Haintz, G. L., Graham, M., & McKenzie, H. (2015). Navigating the ethics of cross-cultural health promotion research. *Health Promotion Journal of Australia, 26*(3), 235–240.

39. Hák, T., Janoušková, S., & Moldan, B. (2016). Sustainable development goals: A need for relevant indicators. *Ecological Indicators, 60*, 565–573.

40. Harrison, T. (2006). Health promotion for persons with disabilities: What does the literature reveal? *Family & Community Health, 29*(1), 12S–19S.

41. Hashemzadeh, M., Rahimi, A., Zare-Farashbandi, F., Alavi-Naeini, A. M., & Daei, A. (2019). Transtheoretical model of health behavioral change: A systematic review. *Iranian Journal of Nursing and Midwifery Research, 24*(2), 83–90.

42. Haugan, G., & Eriksson, M. (2021). An introduction to the health promotion perspective in the health care services. In G. Haugan & M. Eriksson (Eds.), *Health Promotion in Health Care–Vital Theories and Research* (pp. 3–14). Springer.

43. Hawk, C., Ndetan, H., & Evans, Jr. M. W. (2012). Potential role of complementary and alternative health care providers in chronic disease prevention and health promotion: An analysis of National Health Interview Survey data. *Preventive Medicine, 54*(1), 18–22.

44. Head, K. J., Noar, S. M., Iannarino, N. T., & Grant Harrington, N. (2013). Efficacy of text messaging-based interventions for health promotion: A meta-analysis. *Social Science & Medicine, 97*, 41-48.

45. Holtz, C. (2013). *Global Health Care: Issues and Policies.* Jones & Bartlett Learning.

46. Hovell, M. F., Wahlgren, D. R., & Gehrman, C. A. (2002). The behavioral ecological model. In R. J. DiClemente, R. A. Crosby, & M. C. Kegler (Eds.), *Emerging Theories in Health Promotion Practice and Research: Strategies for Improving Public Health* (pp. 347–385). Jossey-Bass.

47. Howse, E., Rychetnik, L., Marks, L., & Wilson, A. (2020). What does the future hold for chronic disease prevention research? *Australian and New Zealand Journal of Public Health, 44*(5), 336–340.
48. Hyman, I., & Guruge, S. (2002). A review of theory and health promotion strategies for new immigrants. *Canadian Journal of Public Health, 93*(3), 183–187.
49. Jackson, S. F., Perkins, F., Khandor, E., Cordwell, L., Hamann, S., & Buasai, S. (2006). Integrated health promotion strategies: A contribution to tackling current and future health challenges. *Health Promotion International, 21*(Suppl_1), 75–83.
50. Janz, N. K., & Becker, M. H. (1984). The health belief model: A decade later. *Health Education Quarterly, 11*(1), 1–47.
51. Kirmayer, L. J. (2012). Rethinking cultural competence. *Transcultural Psychiatry, 49*(2), 149–164.
52. Koelen, M. A., & Van Den Ban, A. W. (2023). *Health Education and Health Promotion*. BRILL.
53. Kokorelias, K. M., Gignac, M. A., Naglie, G., & Cameron, J. I. (2019). Towards a universal model of family centered care: A scoping review. *BMC Health Services Research, 19*(1), 1–11.
54. Krause, T. M., Schaefer, C., & Highfield, L. (2021). The association of social determinants of health with health outcomes. *American Journal of Managed Care, 27*(3), e89–e96.
55. Kumar, S., & Preetha, G. (2012). Health promotion: An effective tool for global health. *Indian Journal of Community Medicine, 37*(1), 5–12.
56. Lando, J., Williams, S. M., Sturgis, S., & Williams, B. (2006). A logic model for the integration of mental health into chronic disease prevention and health promotion. *Preventing Chronic Disease, 3*(2), A61.
57. Landon, B. E., Hicks, L. S., O'Malley, A. J., Lieu, T. A., Keegan, T., McNeil, B. J., & Guadagnoli, E. (2007). Improving the management of chronic disease at community health centers. *New England Journal of Medicine, 356*(9), 921–934.
58. Lee, J. Y. (2012). Future directions for health promotion programs in the public sector. *Korean Journal of Health Education and Promotion, 29*(4), 29–38.
59. Lee, N. R., & Kotler, P. (2015). *Social Marketing: Changing Behaviors for Good* (5th ed.). Sage Publications.
60. Lydia, O. Y. (2019). Social mobilization and community participation in development programmes. *Asian Journal of Social Science, 47*(4), 1–15.
61. Marmot, M., & Wilkinson, R. (2005). *Social Determinants of Health*. Oup Oxford.
62. Martin, G. M., Bergman, A., & Barzilai, N. (2007). Genetic determinants of human health span and life span: Progress and new opportunities. *PLoS Genetics, 3*(7), e125.
63. Mascie-Taylor, C. N., & Karim, E. (2003). The burden of chronic disease. *Science, 302*(5652), 1921, 1922.
64. Mathews, S. C., McShea, M. J., Hanley, C. L., Ravitz, A., Labrique, A. B., & Cohen, A. B. (2019). Digital health: A path to validation. *NPJ Digital Medicine, 2*(1), 38.
65. McKenzie, J. F., Neiger, B. L., & Thackeray, R. (2022). *Planning, Implementing, and Evaluating Health Promotion Programs*. Jones & Bartlett Learning.

66. Miller, A. M., & Iris, M. (2002). Health promotion attitudes and strategies in older adults. *Health Education & Behavior, 29*(2), 249–267.

67. Motola, I., Devine, L. A., Chung, H. S., Sullivan, J. E., & Issenberg, S. B. (2013). Simulation in healthcare education: A best evidence practical guide. AMEE Guide No. 82. *Medical Teacher, 35*(10), e1511–e1530.

68. Murray, C. J., & Lopez, A. D. (2013). Measuring the global burden of disease. *New England Journal of Medicine, 369*(5), 448–457.

69. Peterson, R. A. (1992). Understanding audience segmentation: From elite and mass to omnivore and univore. *Poetics, 21*(4), 243–258.

70. Potvin, L., & Jones, C. M. (2011). Twenty-five years after the Ottawa Charter: The critical role of health promotion for public health. *Canadian Journal of Public Health, 102*, 244-248.

71. Prüss-Ustün, A., Wolf, J., Corvalán, C., Neville, T., Bos, R., & Neira, M. (2017). Diseases due to unhealthy environments: An updated estimate of the global burden of disease attributable to environmental determinants of health. *Journal of Public Health, 39*(3), 464–475.

72. Raphael, D. (2008). Grasping at straws: A recent history of health promotion in Canada. *Critical Public Health, 18*(4), 483–495.

73. Richardson, L. D., & Norris, M. (2010). Access to health and health care: How race and ethnicity matter. *Mount Sinai Journal of Medicine: A Journal of Translational and Personalized Medicine, 77*(2), 166–177.

74. Rimal, R. N., & Lapinski, M. K. (2009). Why health communication is important in public health. *Bulletin of the World Health Organization, 87*, 247–247a.

75. Rodin, J., & Ickovics, J. R. (1990). Women's health: Review and research agenda as we approach the 21st century. *American Psychologist, 45*(9), 1018.

76. Rootman, I. (2001). *Evaluation in Health Promotion: Principles and Perspectives* (No. 92). WHO Regional Office Europe.

77. Ruger, J. P. (2004). Health and social justice. *The Lancet, 364*(9439), 1075–1080.

78. Salazar, L. F., Crosby, R. A., & DiClemente, R. J. (2015). *Research Methods in Health Promotion*. John Wiley & Sons.

79. Scambler, G. (2012). Health inequalities. *Sociology of Health & Illness, 34*(1), 130–146.

80. Schulz, A. J., Krieger, J., & Galea, S. (2002). Addressing social determinants of health: Community-based participatory approaches to research and practice. *Health Education & Behavior, 29*(3), 287–295.

81. Selmani, A., Coenen, M., Voss, S., & Jung-Sievers, C. (2021). Health indices for the evaluation and monitoring of health in children and adolescents in prevention and health promotion: A scoping review. *BMC Public Health, 21*, 1–14.

82. Sheeran, P., Klein, W. M., & Rothman, A. J. (2017). Health behavior change: Moving from observation to intervention. *Annual Review of Psychology, 68*, 573–600.

83. Snyder, L. B. (2007). Health communication campaigns and their impact on behavior. *Journal of Nutrition Education and Behavior, 39*(2), S32–S40.

84. St Leger, L. (2003). Health and nature—New challenges for health promotion. *Health Promotion International, 18*(3), 173–175.

85. Stellefson, M., Paige, S. R., Chaney, B. H., & Chaney, J. D. (2020). Evolving role of social media in health promotion: Updated responsibilities for health education specialists. *International Journal of Environmental Research and Public Health, 17*(4), 1153.

86. Steyn, K., & Damasceno, A. (2006). Lifestyle and related risk factors for chronic diseases. In *Disease and Mortality in Sub-Saharan Africa* (2nd ed., pp. 247–265).

87. Strasser, T., & Gallagher, J. (1994). The ethics of health communication. *World Health Forum, 15*(2), 175–177.

88. Taylor, E., Jantzen, A., & Clow, B. (2013). *Rethinking LGBTQ Health*. Atlantic Centre for Excellence for Women's Health.

89. Terry, N. P., & Francis, L. P. (2007). Ensuring the privacy and confidentiality of electronic health records. *University of Illinois Law Review, 2007*(3), 681–738.

90. Tones, K., & Tilford, S. (2001). *Health Promotion: Effectiveness, Efficiency, and Equity*. Nelson Thornes.

91. Ureda, J., & Yates, S. (2005). A systems view of health promotion. *Journal of Health and Human Services Administration, 28*(1), 5–38.

92. Winett, R. A. (1995). A framework for health promotion and disease prevention programs. *American Psychologist, 50*(5), 341–350.

93. Wold, B., & Mittelmark, M. B. (2018). Health-promotion research over three decades: The social-ecological model and challenges in implementation of interventions. *Scandinavian Journal of Public Health, 46*(20_suppl), 20–26.

94. World Health Organization, (2015). *WHO Recommendations on Health Promotion Interventions for Maternal and Newborn Health 2015*. World Health Organization.

95. World Health Organization, (2020). *Air Quality Guidelines for Europe*. World Health Organization.

96. Zhang, C. Q., Zhang, R., Schwarzer, R., & Hagger, M. S. (2019). A meta-analysis of the health action process approach. *Health Psychology, 38*(7), 623–632.

INDEX

D

E

F

G

H